D1499737

Health in Rural
North America

HEALTH IN RURAL NORTH AMERICA

*The Geography of Health Care
Services and Delivery*

EDITED BY

Wilbert M. Gesler
and
Thomas C. Ricketts

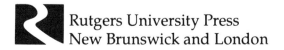

Rutgers University Press
New Brunswick and London

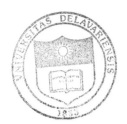

RA
771
.7
.N7
H43
1992

Library of Congress Cataloging-in-Publication Data

Health in rural North America : the geography of health care services and
delivery / edited by Wilbert M. Gesler and Thomas C. Ricketts.
    p.   cm.
Includes bibliographical references and index.
ISBN 0-8135-1759-1 (cloth) ISBN 0-8135-1760-5 (pbk.)
1. Rural health—North America. 2. Medical geography—North America.
I. Gesler, Wilbert M., 1941–   .   II. Ricketts, Thomas C.
RA771.7.N7H43   1992   91-17840
362.1'0425—dc20   CIP

The editors would like to acknowledge the many hours of patient and
painstaking care that Ms. Diana Osborne, Information and Communications
Specialist, Cecil G. Sheps Center for Health Services Research, University of
North Carolina, Chapel Hill, gave to the compilation and editing of this book.
Her attention to numerous but necessary details was essential to its accurate and
timely completion.

Contents

PART THREE: SERVICE PROVISION AND POLICY ISSUES

List of Figures

List of Tables

Contributors

ELIZABETH BELL is a Resident in Anesthesiology in the Medical School, University of North Carolina at Chapel Hill.

ELIZABETH CROMARTIE is a Research Associate at the Health Services Research Center, University of North Carolina at Chapel Hill.

GORDON H. DeFRIESE is Director of the Health Services Research Center, University of North Carolina at Chapel Hill.

WILBERT M. GESLER is Associate Professor of Geography at the University of North Carolina at Chapel Hill.

RENA J. GORDON is Research Assistant Professor in the College of Medicine, University of Arizona, Tucson, and Adjunct Professor in the School of Health Administration and Policy, Arizona State University, Tempe.

MICHAEL R. GREENBERG is Professor of Urban Studies and Community Health at Rutgers University, New Brunswick, New Jersey.

G. BRENT HALL is Associate Professor in the School of Urban and Regional Planning, Faculty of Environmental Studies, University of Waterloo, Waterloo, Ontario.

SUSAN HARTWELL is a Senior Research Associate at Inter-Study, Excelsior, Minnesota.

MARIA HEWITT is a Senior Analyst at the Congressional Office of Technology Assessment, Washington, D.C.

ROBERT G. HUGHES is Research Fellow in the Office of Health Statistics and Analysis, Robert Wood Johnson Foundation, Princeton, New Jersey.

ALUN E. JOSEPH is Professor of Geography and an associate of the Gerontology Research Centre, University of Guelph.

MELINDA S. MEADE is Professor of Geography and a Fellow of the Carolina Population Center, University of North Carolina at Chapel Hill.

JOEL S. MEISTER is Research Assistant Professor in the Rural Health Office of the College of Medicine, University of Arizona, Tucson.

ERIC G. MOORE is Professor and Head of the Department of Geography, Queen's University, Kingston, Ontario.

GEOFFREY B. NELSON is Associate Professor in the Department of Psychology, Wilfrid Laurier University, Waterloo, Ontario.

GREGORY R. NYCZ is Director of Health Systems Research at the Marshfield Medical Research and Education Foundation, a Division of the Marshfield Clinic, Marshfield, Wisconsin.

SYDNEY J. PARLOUR is a recent graduate of the M.A. program in Social-Community Psychology, Wilfrid Laurier University, Waterloo, Ontario.

THOMAS C. RICKETTS is Director of the Rural Health Research Program, Health Services Research Center, University of North Carolina at Chapel Hill.

MARK W. ROSENBERG is an Associate Professor in the Department of Geography, Queen's University, Kingston, Ontario.

ROBERT RUTLEDGE is Assistant Professor in the Department of Surgery, University of North Carolina at Chapel Hill.

JOHN R. SCHMELZER is Senior Researcher for the Wisconsin Rural Health Research Center at the Marshfield Medical Research and Education Foundation, a Division of the Marshfield Clinic, Marshfield, Wisconsin.

DONA SCHNEIDER is Assistant Professor of Urban Studies and Community Health at Rutgers University, New Brunswick, New Jersey.

RICHARD T. WALSH is Assistant Professor and Director of the Social-Community Psychology Program, Department of Psychology, Wilfrid Laurier University, Waterloo, Ontario.

LYNN WHITENER is Librarian at the Health Services Research Center, University of North Carolina at Chapel Hill.

GLENN WILSON is Professor in the Department of Social Medicine, University of North Carolina at Chapel Hill.

Health in Rural
North America

Chapter 1

Introduction

WILBERT M. GESLER, SUSAN HARTWELL,
THOMAS C. RICKETTS, AND
MARK W. ROSENBERG

It is a standard feature of discussions of spatial inequalities in health care delivery to emphasize two areas in which delivery tends to be relatively poor: inner cities and rural areas. Rural areas, the geographic focus of this book, are often described as being peripheral to urban cores in terms of a variety of factors, such as level of economic activity and access to resources. Rural health has long been emphasized by medical geographers and others concerned with the spatial aspects of health care delivery. As an example, the first book-length entry into the North American health care delivery literature (Shannon and Dever, 1974) featured on its cover a sign advertising for a small-town doctor in Ohio.

In recent years, there has been a great amount of discussion about whether medical personnel, physicians in particular, have been moving to rural areas in sufficient numbers to provide adequate health care. There are many problems facing rural health care delivery besides staffing issues, however. Problems of patient accessibility include overcoming relatively long distances to care and inadequate transportation. Many rural hospitals are not financially viable and are being forced to close. New, potentially beneficial, health care options such as health maintenance organizations tend to reach rural areas relatively late. Rural areas contain relatively high proportions of those who need health services the most: the poor, the elderly, blacks, American Indians, and others. The high costs of medical technology often affect rural areas more than urban places.

These issues, and a host of related problems, have been widely discussed in scholarly research and government reports. Much of the work, explicitly or implicitly, has spatial aspects. What is needed now, we feel, is a volume that provides some structure to this wealth of information. To many of us, rural health care problems are seen in very general terms and so they overwhelm us and appear to be intractable. We must bring some specificity to such vague distinctions as "core" and "periphery". We must come to grips with such issues as geographic variability, changes over space in proportions of high-risk groups, and program diffusion. We propose to do this with two main goals in mind: (1) to apply current concepts and techniques of geography and other social sciences to specific problems of health care delivery in rural areas in North America, and (2) to review the literature, develop research frameworks, present case studies, and make policy suggestions about these issues.

The U.S. federal government has manifested an unusual amount of concern with rural health over the past few years. To address this concern, the Office of Rural Health Policy of the Health Resources and Services Administration funded five rural health research centers. The Health Services Research Center (HSRC) of the University of North Carolina at Chapel Hill received one of these grants. Several researchers at HSRC and faculty and graduate students in the department of geography at the University of North Carolina became involved in one particular project developed by the HSRC: a rural health atlas of the United States.

Given the interest at the University of North Carolina, Chapel Hill, in rural health matters, we felt that a climate had been created in which an edited book on current geographic issues in rural health care delivery in North America could be attempted. We contacted those known to be working in this area, and sent out requests for contributions through various channels. The result of this solicitation was, as anticipated, not a complete coverage of all the major problems facing rural health care in North America today, but certainly a set of chapters that cover a wide variety of pertinent issues. Since the Canadian contribution to the geography of rural health care has been both significant and substantial, we were pleased to receive three contributions from north of the border. Thus we draw attention to "North America" in the book's title. Although the medical care systems and current concerns of Canada and the United States are quite different in many ways, problems such as costs and geographic isolation are common. We have made attempts, where appropriate, to compare and contrast the two countries within the North American region.

In the remainder of this chapter we will set the stage for the rest of the book by providing an overview of the history of rural health care in North America, discussing some major aspects of the current rural environment, giving a brief overview of some key issues in rural health care, previewing the chapters to follow, and emphasizing the geographic concepts and methodologies used by the various contributors.

Historical Overview of Rural Health Care in the United States

Before beginning a discussion of the issues now facing rural health care providers, it is worthwhile to examine important historical developments that have shaped the present rural health care climate.

In the early years of white settlement in North America, most physicians were individual practitioners who provided the full range of medical services needed by their patients. As generalists, they delivered whatever services the available technology could support. In 1910, a significant development occurred in the United States that shaped the future delivery of medical care—namely, the dissemination of the Flexner Report on medical education. Among the many changes fostered by this report was greater differentiation into medical specialties. Because of the need to train specialists in clinical settings where there were large numbers of patients, increasing numbers of physicians began to be concentrated in urban areas. By the 1930s, this trend had progressed far enough to trigger alarm about physician distribution and patients' access to services in rural areas.

Later in the 1930s, the financial distress caused by the Depression resulted in the U.S. federal government becoming involved in financing direct general medical services for the first time. Through the Farm Security Administration (FSA), the government provided prepaid health service for low-income and economically marginal farm families. By 1942, the FSA was serving 600,000 people in 1,100 rural counties, with an additional 150,000 receiving care through its migrant farm worker program (Murrin, 1982).

Although this program was phased out after World War II, it established an important precedent for the involvement of the federal government in financing health care services.

Another noteworthy development resulting from the Depression was the proliferation of nonprofit Blue Cross and Blue Shield insurance plans during the 1940s. By spreading the costs of care over a broad population, these plans made health care services much more affordable for many people. Since self-employed farmers and employees of small businesses could not be readily enrolled in groups, however, nonmetropolitan communities were affected by these plans to a far lesser degree than urban areas. Nonetheless, the introduction of third-party insurance coverage was a significant event on the rural health care scene.

After World War II, the federal government assumed an important role in shaping the delivery of rural health care through the passage of the Hospital Survey and Construction Act of 1946. This act, usually referred to as the Hill-Burton program, consisted of heavy federal investment in the construction and modernization of nonfederal health care facilities. Between 1947 and 1962, Hill-Burton funds were used in 30 percent of all hospital construction projects. Significantly, nearly 40 percent of the projects funded under Hill-Burton were initiated in communities with populations under 10,000. The impact of the program on rural communities was immense, as the federal government spent a total of $3.7 billion on the construction of nonprofit community hospitals between 1947 and 1971 (Murrin, 1982).

A major outcome of the Hill-Burton program was a significant improvement in the quality of health care in rural areas. Prior to Hill-Burton, most hospitals in rural communities had been small, proprietary facilities that did not meet accepted standards of acute care. With Hill-Burton funds, many of these antiquated facilities were replaced with modern, well-equipped community hospitals.

A secondary objective of the Hill-Burton program was to attract physicians to rural areas by increasing their access to high-quality acute care facilities. Since the physician distribution problem was already a concern to many health planners, it was hoped that the technology and modern conveniences made possible by Hill-Burton would make rural communities more attractive to physicians. Regrettably, the hoped-for redistribution did not occur, and the distribution of physicians in fact worsened, as other factors still held sway in their choice of practice location.

Concern over the rural physician shortage became particularly acute in the late 1960s and early 1970s. Although the number of physicians in patient care had increased from 119 per 100,000 population in 1950 to 137 per 100,000 in 1970, the disparity between urban and rural areas in 1970 was, respectively, 192 physicians per 100,000 versus 41. Furthermore, there were 50 percent fewer general practitioners in rural areas in 1970 than in 1930 (Coleman, 1976). Those who remained tended to be older and often were not replaced with new physicians upon retirement.

To help counteract this alarming trend, several important federal legislative initiatives were introduced beginning in 1964. In that year, the Office of Economic Opportunity funded the Neighborhood Health Centers program to provide ambulatory care in rural and inner-city areas. The Rural Health Initiative (RHI), introduced in 1975, reflected the federal government's desire to consolidate the previously disjointed rural health programs into a coherent approach for meeting rural health care needs.

A component of the RHI, originally a Medicaid demonstration program, was the Health Underserved Rural Areas (HURA) program. This initiative consisted of innovative research and demonstration efforts designed to explore new ways of providing care for remote rural populations. Many of these projects were oriented toward enhancing physicians' impact through the use of nurse practitioners and physicians' assistants. HURA, in conjunction with the Primary Care Research and Development Program, achieved a measure of success in making primary care more available to people in rural communities.

Another major attempt to alleviate the effects of physician maldistribution came in the form of several pieces of health personnel legislation in the 1970s. The National Health Service Corps (NHSC) was launched in 1970 under the Emergency Health Personnel Act. Through the NHSC, medical students received loan forgiveness in exchange for serving in designated areas considered to have physician shortages. Through subsequent health professions legislation medical schools were encouraged to enroll more students electing primary care specialties. This provision stipulated that a medical school receive a fixed grant for each student as long as the school increased its annual enrollment and maintained a specified percentage of first-year residencies in primary care specialties.

As originally stipulated, shortage areas were identified as those with a primary care physician-to-population ratio of less than 1 : 4,000. Since the use of the basic population ratios made it difficult to assess shortage areas validly, more extensive shortage criteria were stipulated in the Health Professions Education Assistance Act of 1976. The new criteria still included a population ratio, though the acceptable minimum was raised to one physician per 3,500 population. In addition, the criteria also included standards for rates of poverty, fertility, and infant mortality. Certain groups, including Native Americans and migrant laborers, were designated as needy solely on the basis of their unique problems in accessing care. Starting in 1981, NHSC administrators tried to target Corps placements to areas of greatest need using the High Impact Placement Opportunity List. By 1987, 65 percent of all Corps placements were in rural areas. Although many rural areas have benefited by having Corps placements where otherwise there might have been *no* providers, some policy-makers feel the program has relieved rural communities from the responsibility of recruiting their own physicians. Now, with the recent decline in financial support for the NHSC, the availability of Corps physicians is much more limited than ever before.

Despite the determined efforts of the federal government to promote better physician distribution, most experts agree that the results of these initiatives were disappointing. The poorest results were achieved in sparsely populated and remote counties. According to Langwell et al. (1985), only 21 percent of nonmetropolitan counties (see chapter 2 for definitions of nonmetropolitan and metropolitan counties) with populations less than 10,000 added even one new physician between 1975 and 1979, even though this was the period when federal efforts were most intense. In contrast, 40 percent of *all* nonmetropolitan counties gained at least one physician.

Historical Overview of Rural
Health Care in Canada

Constitutionally, Canadian health care is in the domain of the provincial governments. Historically, this means that each province has defined its own health care system. It also means that the role of the Canadian federal government has been to try to insure

uniformity of health care programs among the provincial governments by using cost-sharing agreements as "carrots" and "sticks"
at various times since World War II.

In the early part of the twentieth century Canada lagged behind
the United States in developing social legislation in general, and
health care legislation in particular (Naylor, 1986; Torrance, 1987).
Although government commissions were appointed and legislation proposed, the first universal hospital insurance program was
not created until after World War II. In 1947, the province of
Saskatchewan, under the Co-operative Commonwealth Federation Party (forerunner of the New Democratic Party), enacted the
first legislation in what was, and continues to be, a province
dominated by a rural economy.

The Saskatchewan initiative was followed in 1948 by the Federal Health Grants program, whose main purpose was to help
provincial governments build and renovate hospitals that had
been neglected during the Depression and war years (Torrance,
1987, 24). During the 1950s some provincial governments followed the Saskatchewan lead, but there was tremendous variation in the level of coverage and the criteria set for eligibility. As
a result, in 1957, the Canadian federal government passed the
Hospital Insurance and Diagnostics Act. The heart of this legislation was the intent of the federal government to share the
costs of hospital care with the provinces, a step that created
provincial hospital insurance, universally available to all residents of the province. Through the late 1950s and 1960s, provincial governments first created hospital insurance programs, and
then some also instituted insurance programs to cover physician costs outside the hospital.

In response to the myriad of provincial programs, disparities in
health status by region as well as by income, and disparities in the
level of health services and expenditures by provinces, in 1961 the
Royal Commission on Health Services (often referred to as the
Hall Commission, after its head, Justice Emmett Hall) was formed
to examine Canada's health care system in its entirety. What resulted in 1964 was a multivolume report and a recommendation
for universal and comprehensive health insurance for the Canadian population. These recommendations were translated into
federal legislation in the 1968 Medical Care Act, which provided
federal financial support to provinces that implemented the principles of the Medical Care Act. In a few short years, every province

had either adopted their existing plans or developed plans to create universal and comprehensive health insurance.

Each step taken to move from an essentially private, market-driven health care system to one essentially state-based was contested by various groups, but especially the provincial and national medical associations, the private health insurance industry, and conservative political parties, at least until the early 1960s (see Naylor, 1986; Taylor, 1987a; Torrance, 1987). It is also worth noting that the Medical Care Act allowed provincial governments substantial latitude to define what services would be covered and how physicians would be remunerated under their provincial health care plans.

The issue of physician remuneration led the Canadian federal government to intervene one more time in the 1980s. As the result of yet another federal study by Justice Hall, the Canadian federal government passed the Canada Health Act in 1984. One of its purposes was to convince provincial governments to do away with physician remuneration practices the Canadian federal government felt were deterring accessibility to health care.

There is no doubt that the cumulative effects of provincial and federal legislation contributed to the creation of more hospital beds (Taylor, 1987a) and greater overall economic access to health care among the Canadian population (Manga, 1987). What is not so clear are the impacts on low-income individuals and families, and on rural compared to urban individuals and families.

In the late 1970s, life expectancy for people with the lowest income level was 71.9 years, compared to 76.4 years for those in the highest-income group, and people living in the smallest communities (less than 1,000 population) and rural areas had life expectancies of 72.5 years, compared to 75.3 years for people living in cities with populations over one million (Wilkens and Adams, 1987, 49).

Although the population-per-physician ratio has improved steadily since the 1950s (Taylor, 1987b), in Canada as a whole and in every province, there remain substantial differences in ratios between the larger and more urban provinces and the smaller and more rural provinces. Most studies of population-per-physician ratios carried out at the subprovincial level indicate that there are absolute differences between urban and rural geographic units and that the relative disparities have remained constant over time (Anderson and Rosenberg, 1990; Northcott, 1980; Spaulding and Spitzer, 1972; Thrall and

Tsitanidis, 1983). Virtually every province has recognized this issue and has some form of program to encourage physicians to practice in rural areas. The success of these programs in addressing rural inequalities in population-per-physician ratios is, however, questionable (Anderson and Rosenberg, 1990).

The Current Rural Environment in the United States

One cannot analyze the problems now being encountered in rural health care except by looking at the larger rural environment. The prevailing demographic, economic, and social conditions in rural America have had a substantial impact on how health care services are delivered. This section will provide an overview of some aspects of the rural environment, including occupational and income information, health status indicators, and utilization statistics. Other important components of the rural situation—including population characteristics, health insurance coverage, physician shortages, and accessibility—will be covered in later chapters.

Without a doubt, the *occupational* profile of metropolitan and nonmetropolitan areas has changed dramatically in the last half-century. Most notably, the proportion of persons engaged in farming occupations has declined significantly. In 1920, 30 percent of the total population lived on farms; by 1950, this figure had declined to 15 percent; by 1984, it stood at 2.4 percent (Wimberly, 1986). Even more illustrative of the overall trend away from farming is the changing residence distribution *within* the rural population. In 1920, 61 percent of all rural residents were farm dwellers, while by 1984, only 9 percent of rural residents lived on farms (Wimberly, 1986). Although these figures do not reflect the number of individuals actually engaged in farming as an occupation, they provide a reasonably accurate proxy. Table 1.1 shows the distribution of occupations in metropolitan and nonmetropolitan areas. Clearly, the tertiary sector (with the exception of relatively low-paying service jobs) is overrepresented in metro areas, whereas the primary and secondary sectors are over-represented in nonmetropolitan areas.

Rural areas have long been *economically* disadvantaged relative to their urban counterparts. Since 1965, rural per capita income has ranged from 69 to 77 percent of urban income. In

Table 1.1. Economic and Health Status Indicators by
Nonmetropolitan and Metropolitan Counties

	Nonmetropolitan	Metropolitan
Occupation (percent employed)		
Managerial and professional	17.2	25.4
Technical, sales, administrative	24.1	32.7
Operators, fabricators, laborers	21.0	14.4
Service	14.5	13.2
Precision, production, craft, repair	14.0	12.2
Farming, forestry, fishing	9.3	2.1
Self-assessed health status (percent)		
Excellent	35.8	40.6
Very good	26.1	27.5
Good	24.9	22.5
Fair	9.4	6.8
Poor	3.9	2.6

Sources: Beale and Fuguitt (1985), National Center for Health Statistics (1986b).

1984, the average per capita income in rural counties was $10,000, a mere 71 percent of the $14,000 urban average (American Hospital Association, 1987). Similar disparities have been identified for the over-65 population, as a 1985 analysis showed the median income of farm and nonfarm elders to be, respectively, 71 percent and 65 percent of urban elders' income (Goudy and Dobson, 1988).

It should be noted that there is considerable disparity in incomes among the various types of rural counties (see chapter 2 on county classifications). Rural counties that depend on farming, mining, and manufacturing are lagging substantially behind metropolitan counties, whereas those characterized by retirement settlements and government installations are keeping pace and in some cases exceeding metropolitan income growth (Cordes, 1987). As might be expected, the income profile of a thriving retirement county also differs markedly from that of a persistent poverty county in which the major economic base is subsistence agriculture. This vast diversity in the economic status of rural counties makes it difficult to develop national responses to rural health care problems.

Another useful indicator of economic status is the rate of poverty among the urban and rural populations. It is significant to note that eighty-five of the eighty-six persistent poverty counties in the nation are located in rural areas (*Rural Aging Roundup*, 1987). Overall poverty rates in rural areas have traditionally exceeded those in urban areas. In 1985, 18.3 percent of the rural population (all ages) fell below the federal poverty level, while only 13.8 percent of the urban population was classified as impoverished (Cordes, 1987). One of the explanations for the observed income differences between metropolitan and nonmetropolitan counties pertains to underemployment. In 1982, 18.1 percent of nonmetropolitan workers were underemployed, versus 12.3 percent of workers in metropolitan areas. The unemployment profile is not as distinctive, as the 1982 nonmetropolitan unemployment rate was 8.0 percent, compared to 6.8 percent in metropolitan areas.

Unquestionably, economic conditions in nonmetropolitan areas have deteriorated significantly in recent years. In the early 1980s, increased international production of agricultural and energy products decreased the demand for these goods. In addition, high interest rates and falling land values caused substantial difficulties for farmers, and, as a result, for the rural businesses supported by their purchases. The timber and mining industries have also suffered economic hardships owing to the diminshed demand for new homes, automobiles, and other goods (American Hospital Association, 1989).

Both historical and recent evidence suggests that rural residents have more serious and severe *health problems* than their urban counterparts (see chapter 3 for a discussion of rural/urban differences in mortality rates and for the effect of poverty on these rates). These problems are often compounded by poverty, poor nutrition, substandard housing, occupational hazards, transportation difficulties, and limited medical resources.

Many of the studies on health status rely on patient self-reporting rather than clinical indicators or functional assessments. This is due in large part to the methodological difficulties encountered in collecting empirical data on health status. As shown in table 1.1, metropolitan residents surveyed in 1985 were somewhat more likely to report excellent or very good health status, while nonmetropolitan residents more frequently indicated that their health status was only good, fair, or poor.

Some of the reasons suggested for the rural/urban discrepancy in health status include the prevalence of more hazardous and strenuous work activities in rural areas, limited access to health care, and insufficient financial means for purchasing health services. In a study of federal Health Manpower Shortage Areas, residents of those areas were found less likely to have visited a physician in the previous year and more likely to report fair or poor health status. The study was not conclusive, however, as to whether these differences were purely a function of residence status, or whether they could be attributed to income and insurance differences between shortage and nonshortage areas (Berk et al., 1983).

Research findings indicate that nonmetropolitan residents experience a *greater* incidence of chronic illness than metropolitan residents, but a *lesser* incidence of acute illness. This disparity in the incidence of acute illnesses is not substantial, as a 1985 survey showed there to be 178 acute conditions per 100 persons per year in metropolitan areas, versus 166 for nonmetropolitan counties (U.S. National Center for Health Statistics, 1986a). When studies are controlled for the differing urban/rural incidence, however, rural residents who have acute illnesses are *less* likely to report restricted activity, disability days, or loss of work than are acutely ill urban residents (U.S. National Center for Health Statistics, 1986b). One can only speculate as to the reasons why, but the finding may be related to the nature of rural residents' occupations, their lack of traditional sick-day benefits, or cultural attitudes toward work (see chapter 7 for more on the possible effects of rural cultural attitudes on health status). For example, a self-employed farmer will likely continue working through all but the most serious health conditions in order to take care of the crops and protect the family's future livelihood.

Research on chronic illness indicates that persons residing in rural areas are more commonly afflicted with the following *chronic* conditions: arthritis, visual and hearing impairments, ulcers, thyroid and kidney problems, heart disease, hypertension, and emphysema (U.S. National Center for Health Statistics, 1986b). Unlike the findings for acute conditions, rural residents are slightly more likely to suffer activity restrictions because of chronic conditions than are urban dwellers (U.S. National Center for Health Statistics, 1986b). These findings corroborate the analyses of Berk et al. (1984). The greater incidence of chronic illness in rural areas may be partly explained by the higher proportion of elderly residents (see chapter 4 on the implications of changing demographic structures for rural health care).

Recent research findings on the *utilization* of health care services by urban and rural residents are somewhat contradictory. Much of the earlier research indicated that persons living in rural areas utilize fewer health services than their urban counterparts. The causes for this disparity are complex, but contributing factors include the greater likelihood of being uninsured, the limited availability of providers, and substantial travel distance to service locations (Berk et al., 1983).

One portion of the research on utilization has focused on rural residents' access to and use of *physician* services (chapter 8 discusses this issue in detail, with a focus on why there are physician shortages in certain areas) (U.S. National Center for Health Statistics, 1986b). Slightly higher percentages of the nonmetropolitan population under age 65 (29.0%) had no physician visits in 1984 compared to a similar metropolitan population (26.8%). However, insurance coverage seemed to be a stronger determinant than residence of whether or not a person received physician care; those with Medicaid had lower proportions of no physican visits (17.2%) than those with private insurance (25.9%) or the uninsured (40.8%). It should be noted that the propensity of rural residents to travel to urban areas for health care has increased in recent years, thus making it more likely for people to receive services even if they are not available in their local community. One reason for this increased mobility is the improvement in road quality; another is residents' increasing likelihood of traveling outside the local community to purchase other goods and services. Similar findings were observed with respect to *frequency* of physician visits. In general, rural residents averaged slightly fewer physician visits than urban residents; however, this difference was minimal among the uninsured populations. Once again, the greatest utilization was incurred by Medicaid beneficiaries, followed by those with private insurance coverage and then by the uninsured.

A series of recent studies by the Robert Wood Johnson Foundation suggests that the long-standing disparity in access to physician care between rural and urban areas is narrowing. In 1978, rural farm dwellers were less likely than urban residents to see a physician (Robert Wood Johnson Foundation, 1978). By 1982, rural residents still had a lower average number of physician visits per year, but the gap had nearly closed (Robert Wood Johnson Foundation, 1983). A 1986 survey showed that rural respondents had a mean of 4.4 physician visits per year, compared to 4.3 for urban respondents (Freeman et al., 1987). Some researchers suggest that this improvement may be linked to improvement in rural physician-to-population ratios, as well as to an increase in coverage of rural residents by health insurance.

In contrast to the findings on physician utilization, studies on the use of *hospital* services suggest that rural residents are hospitalized proportionately more frequently than urban residents. Rural persons have an average of 12 hospital episodes per 100 persons, compared to 10 hospital episodes per 100 urban persons (U.S. National Center for Health Statistics, 1984). In the same vein, the 1986 Robert Wood Johnson survey indicated that 8 percent of rural residents had been hospitalized during the preceding year, compared to 6 percent of urban residents (Freeman et al., 1987). The rural/urban disparity is most pronounced between the respective Medicaid populations. In particular, rural nonfarm residents with Medicaid coverage had more hospital episodes than those in any other insurance or residence category. The disparity in rural and urban hospital utilization is somewhat puzzling in view of other rural utilization trends. A contributing explanation might be that, since rural patients are less likely to be under the care of a physician, they may be more ill by the time they receive care, thus necessitating hospitalization.

The Current Rural Environment in Canada

According to the 1986 Census of Canada, 5,957,245 people or 23.5 percent of the population lived in rural areas. Only 890,490 people or 3.5 percent of the total population are classified as living in rural farm areas. The remaining 5,066,755 people in rural Canada are classified as living in rural nonfarm areas.

In 1985, average total income for the farm population was $12,429, compared to $15,980 in the nonfarm population (Beyrouti and Dion, 1990, 23). Among farm families, 3 percent had a negative total income, with losses averaging around $18,000, and about 45 percent had incomes of less than $25,000 (Beyrouti and Dion, 1990, 28).

Although regionally disaggregated data on rural families were not available, contrasts can be drawn between provinces such as Ontario, which are highly urbanized, and provinces such as Newfoundland or Saskatchewan, where the populations are mainly employed in agriculture, fishing, mining, or forestry. For example, in 1987, the unemployment rate in Ontario was 6.1 percent compared to 18.6 percent in Newfoundland or 7.3 percent in Saskatchewan (Statistics Canada, 1989, 5-22).

Rural parts of Canada have been afflicted with the same kinds of problems as have occurred in the rural United States over the past ten years. High interest rates, low prices for natural resources on international markets, and changing technology have meant that the number of people who are employed in these sectors has been declining. Between 1981 and 1987, the percentage change in the number of people employed in agriculture was –3.9 percent; in forestry, the percentage change was –8.3 percent; in mining it was –29.5 percent (Statistics Canada, 1989, 5-22).

Although the connections among environment, lifestyle, socioeconomic status, employment, and morbidity and mortality are complex (see D'Arcy and Siddique, 1987), measures of disability-free life expectancy and quality-adjusted life expectancy are lower for people living in rural Canada than for those in Canada's largest cities. In the late 1970s, the disability-free life expectancy of people living in rural Canada was 60.1 years compared to 64.0 years in cities with populations of over one million, and quality-adjusted life expectancy was 67.4 years in rural Canada compared to 70.6 years in cities of over one million (Wilkens and Adams, 1987, 49).

Finally, it is worth noting two additional groups that generate unique problems for the delivery of health care in rural Canada. In Atlantic Canada, Manitoba and Saskatchewan, and in many other rural parts of Canada as well, depopulation of working-age cohorts has left many communities where the relative percentage of the elderly is very high, although, in absolute terms, they may only number in the hundreds (see Moore et al., 1989).

The second group is the native peoples of Canada, who live mainly in isolated settlements in rural Canada, but primarily in the north. Differences in morbidity and mortality rates between native peoples and the nonnative population and the poor quality of health care delivery for native peoples are well documented (Grescoe, 1987; Lithwick et al., 1986; O'Neil, 1987; Young, 1987). If health care status and delivery are to improve overall in rural Canada, then the special needs of these two groups will have to be addressed in a concrete but sensitive fashion.

Overview of the Book

The book is divided into three sections. The first section, Background, sets the stage by defining the complex notion of rurality, discussing trends in mortality rates, and outlining the potential impact of demographic changes. Part Two, High-Risk Populations, consists of three contributions that address the problems of the provision of in-home health services, providing health services for the disabled, and health care provision for mentally ill children. The third section consists of five chapters that deal with service provision and policy issues: shortages of rural physicians, rural primary care programs, the rural hospital crisis, emergency medical services, and inequalities in health care expenditures.

Anyone embarking on a study of rural health care in North America is immediately confronted with an apparently simple but in reality complex definitional problem: what is rural? Clearly, individual perceptions of what is rural are not sufficiently accurate; perceptions differ and the distinctions societies or individuals make between country and city and the images they convey vary over time (Williams, 1973). However, distinctions do have to be made, based on the purposes of the research and on the data available. In chapter 2, Maria Hewitt tackles the question of what is rural head on. She notes that clear definitions are required as a basis for informed policy decisions, and that these decisions are vital to the health of various groups of people. She then proceeds to compare the rural/urban dichotomy of the Bureau of the Census and the use of metropolitan statistical areas and nonmetropolitan areas by the Office of Management and Budget; to detail the extremely important idea that there is great diversity within rural areas; to discuss the availability and use by federal agencies of health statistics for nonmetropolitan and rural areas; and to critique the strengths and weaknesses of various rural definitions and classifications.

Earlier in this chapter, we explored briefly the relative health status of rural and urban populations, noting in very general terms that rural areas had higher rates of morbidity for some conditions, while urban areas had higher rates for others. Dona Schneider and Michael Greenberg pursue the question of urban/ rural health differentials much further in chapter 3. They first state that, although rural mortality rates were lower earlier in the century in the United States many (but not all) regional death rates have been converging toward national rates; this suggests that a *rural penalty* has now taken the place of the former *urban penalty* for health. The authors test a specific hypothesis, namely that poverty is more important than urbanization in influencing mortality rates. Using age-adjusted death rates for nine major causes of death for white males and females thirty-five to sixty-four years old in selected states from 1939 to 1981, the hypothesis is confirmed to a striking degree. The authors discuss the importance to rural health of several variables related to poverty, including diet, living conditions, personal risk-taking behavior, educational levels, unemployment rates, perceived health status, and access to care.

Associations between need for health services and demographic variables (age, sex, ethnicity, and migration) are well known, but are not always given the attention they deserve in health care planning. Furthermore, demographic structures show great variability across rural areas. Melinda Meade makes and illustrates these important points in chapter 4. The chapter begins by detailing the morbidity and mortality patterns associated with various stages of life—infancy, childhood, young adulthood, maturity, seniority, and old age—and emphasizes that in the future these associations might change. Then spatial variations among counties and states in demographic structure, created by such factors as differential aging, migration from and to metropolitan areas, and fertility behavior, are discussed. The chapter closes with a very useful demographic typology of rural counties—aging, previous out-migration, booming, and retirement destination—illustrated with appropriate county population pyramids.

Since the proportion of elderly is growing in the entire North American population and at a faster rate in rural than in urban areas, great concern has been expressed over health care for the rural elderly. One very important option for addressing growing demands for medical services is in-home care, the subject of Alun Joseph's contribution, chapter 5. In dealing with this topic the author develops a research framework based on some very useful dichotomies—congregation versus concentration of the elderly;

aging in place versus in-migration, and in-home services versus institutional support—and demonstrates the implications of elderly migration and service coordination for health care provision. Two case studies carried out in rural Ontario provide data that complement the research framework; specifically, they deal with a migration typology, service utilization, and a centralized-decentralized One-Stop Access case management pilot project.

Just as it is difficult to define what is rural, so it is often hard to define precisely certain groups in need of health care and other social services. One such group is the disabled, the topic of chapter 6, by Mark Rosenberg and Eric Moore. The authors of this chapter first present information on the scope of the problem and then develop a research agenda for studying the disabled that consists of three parts: defining and measuring disability, the rights of the disabled, and service alternatives. It becomes clear that definitional, legal, and service provision matters concerning the disabled are complex and that the issues underlying them are made even more difficult by the geographic dispersal of the disabled and the lack of financial resources in rural areas. An added feature of this chapter is the parallel description of the disability problem in both Canada and the United States.

Since health care delivery efforts are usually focused on large groups of people such as the elderly or dramatic issues such as AIDS, several groups who are just as much in need of attention tend to fall by the wayside. Brent Hall, Syd Parlour, Geoffrey Nelson, and Richard Walsh focus attention in chapter 7 on one such group, children in need of mental health care. Combining insights from geography and psychology, the authors examine the subject using an ecological framework that is based on three systems—geosocial, sociocultural, and planning, policy, and service delivery—that comprise the context of children's mental health. Ecological notions of interdependence, cycling of resources, adaptation, and succession are also introduced into the discussion. A preliminary analysis of children's mental health in rural northern Ontario and a comparison with the situation in more urbanized southern Ontario suggest that ecological conditions in the former area do not augur well for the mental health of children there.

A great deal has been written and various opinions have been expressed about a major resource concern, imbalance in the supply of physicians between rural and urban areas within North

American health care systems. There has been debate in recent years, for example, about the impact of increases on physician supply on rural places. The issue is complex, to say the least. In chapter 8, Rena Gordon, Robert Hughes, and Joel Meister pull together the voluminous literature on physician shortages and reasons for them into a comprehensible whole by employing a framework based on both a push/pull dichotomy and four scales of analysis: individual, community, state, and national. The chapter thus presents an integrated picture of those factors that may either attract or dissuade physicians to or from practice in rural areas, and of programs and policies that attempt to ameliorate the problem. To provide concreteness, examples from Arizona and other states are discussed to illustrate the utility of the framework.

The attempt to provide primary health care to underserved areas has taken many organizational forms and has evolved and adapted in response to recent political and economic changes in various ways. Using the results of the National Evaluation of Rural Primary Care Programs, Thomas Ricketts and Elizabeth Cromartie examine, in chapter 9, how forty rural primary health care clinics in the United States, all born in subsidy and representing five organizational types, fared between the years 1977 and 1989. Their assessment includes adjustments to competition and financial constraints, program stability, access to care, characteristics of providers, the role of the National Health Service Corps, changes in funding sources, service areas and populations served, and program operation. The authors conclude that, although some rural communities may be losing control over their clinics, most programs have survived and remain community-oriented. Also, several programs have demonstrated an ability for innovative adaptation that shows potential promise for the future viability of rural health programs.

In chapter 10, Gordon DeFriese, Glenn Wilson, Thomas Ricketts, and Lynn Whitener tackle one of the most prominent issues in rural health care, hospital closures. It is well known that there have been alarmingly high rates of rural hospital closures in recent years and also a potential for many more to either close their doors or operate on a different basis in the future. The authors of this chapter discuss the factors that may be responsible for the rural hospital crisis, including, among others, problems related to the Medicare program, demographic changes, the nature of primary care services, and financial margins. Following a literature review of studies of hospital closures, geographic considerations, and studies of hospital consumer behavior, and a review of policy options (which include restructuring individual hospitals, integrating rural facilities, and conversions both within and between levels of care), the authors propose a framework for a national study of the rural hospital situation. The study focuses on a perceived omission in the existing literature and the debate on policy options, namely the views of health care consumers on the utility of existing hospitals and preferences for a wide range of alternatives.

As Robert Rutledge, Thomas Ricketts, and Elizabeth Bell point out in chapter 11, many of the problems faced in rural health care can be seen very clearly in the provision of emergency medical services, and of trauma care in particular. These difficulties include problems in reaching populations dispersed over wide areas, often with inadequate transportation, in time to save lives; relatively poor communications networks; limitations on the availability of trained personnel and on adequate field experience for them; fragmented financing systems; and the inability of many small, rural hospitals to handle emergency cases. To deal with these problems, the authors discuss in detail the use of trauma scores, triaging to direct patients to either trauma centers or non–trauma center hospitals, the use of helicopters for some cases, an integrated systems approach, regionalization of services for greater efficiency, more emphasis on adequate training of personnel, and better financial arrangements for service provision and evaluation.

Everyone is aware of the rapid rise in health care costs and many complain that increased expenditures have not been justified in terms of outcomes. Federal cost-containment efforts, including recent Medicare legislation, are the subject of much current debate; and payment issues have become increasingly prominent in discussions of rural health care. Gregory Nycz and John Schmelzer address the implications of expenditures for rural health in chapter 12. Included in their discussion are the various sources of payment and methods of financing, the role of the federal government, spatial payment inequities, and the two components of Medicare financing. They map out the spatial distribution of adjusted average per capita costs for aged Medicare beneficiaries across U.S. regions and regional subdivisions, based on both economic and metropolitan proximity differentials, and they find clear patterns of spatial inequality. Then they suggest factors that might explain these differences; these include geographic variations in physician and hospital payment rates, need and demand for medical care, supply of providers and facilities, and local medical practice styles.

Geographic Themes

Since this volume is a geography of rural health, it is worth emphasizing the geographic concepts and methodologies employed by the contributors, be they geographers or not. This brief section is particularly addressed to the nongeographers among our readers, who may not be familiar with geographic perspectives. Examples of chapters that illustrate various geographic ideas will be indicated in parentheses throughout the discussion.

One of the principal concerns of the geographic study of health care is the *spatial arrangement* or *distribution* of the various components of health care systems, such as facilities, personnel, and consumers. A particular focus is on the impact of various spatial arrangements on the interactions among system components. Spatial interactions are one of the major components of the availability, accessibility, and utilization of health care resources. Several interrelated approaches, all illustrated in this book, can be taken to analyze spatial distributions and interactions. Determining where client populations, medical personnel, and medical facilities are *located* in relation to each other is clearly important (chapters 5, 8, 9). In rural areas, the *degree of isolation* of health care system components is often of great concern (chapters 2, 7, 11). Much emphasis has been placed in the geographic literature on the *distance* between consumers and providers, measured in a variety of ways, including map distance, road distance, travel time, and travel costs (chapters 2, 6, 8, 10, 11, 12). Obviously, *mode of transport* and *access to transportation* are crucial factors affecting distance (chapters 6, 9, 11). The overall pattern of spatial configurations is of interest as well. Here we encounter discussions of the degree to which a health care system is or should be *centralized* or *decentralized* (chapter 5), what *levels of service* are provided at which *places* and over what *market areas* (chapter 8, 10), and the ways in which health care problems and treatment resources can be *regionalized* (chapters 2, 3, 4, 11).

A second major set of geographic themes that runs throughout the book is the role of the *social, cultural, demographic, political, and economic environments* in which rural health care is delivered. It is granted that this discussion stretches far beyond the bounds of strictly geographic concerns into several other areas of the social science of health. Nonetheless, the interaction between humans and the environment, no matter how widely defined that environment might be, is one of the core traditions in geography. Thus the geographic perspective often examines health care environments in *ecological* terms (chapter 7). There is a recognition that health care delivery systems and their environments *change, evolve,* and *adapt* to new situations over time, just as ecosystems do (chapters 3, 4, 9). An aspect of the environment or *context* of health care that has received special attention by medical geographers and others in recent years is *political economy*, which includes assessing government health care policies at different levels and *spatial inequalities* in service delivery (chapters 3, 5, 6, 9, 12). *Cultural* factors are also highlighted by some contributors (chapters 3, 7, 10).

The third theme cluster that deserves special mention is the tension between two opposites, *spatial regularity* or *pattern* and *spatial diversity* or *uniqueness*. On the one hand, geographic analysis reveals similarities across space, for example in factors associated with physician location (chapter 8) or in third-party payments (chapter 12). In contrast, several contributors stress that health care planners need to recognize the wide variety of local health care systems and environments that exist in rural areas (chapters 2, 4, 5, 10, 12). Partly at issue here is the *scale* of analysis; pattern and diversity manifest themselves at different geographic scales (chapters 4, 6, 7).

To conclude this section, we make the point that, despite the core emphasis on geographic aspects of rural health care, there has been a conscious effort throughout the book to reach out and incorporate nongeographic components. It is a truism to say that no one discipline can adequately express or analyze the complexities of health care delivery.

PART ONE

BACKGROUND

Chapter 2

Defining "Rural" Areas
Impact on Health Care Policy and Research

MARIA HEWITT

Although there has been widespread concern regarding a "health care crisis" in rural areas, there is little agreement as to what rural areas are. How rural areas (or rural populations) are defined is far from academic, since urban/rural designations are basic to participation in certain federal programs and to payment rates from federal sources. Indeed, the perceived magnitude of rural health care problems and the impact of any change in public policy depend on how "rural" is defined.

The features most intuitively associated with rurality are small populations, sparse settlement, and remoteness or distance from large urban settlements. Historically, rural populations have been distinguished from urban ones by their dependence on farming occupations and by differences in family size, lifestyle, and politics (Gilford et al., 1981). However, because of dramatic improvements in transportation and communication, migration to and from rural areas, and diversification of the rural economy, these clear distinctions no longer exist. The presence of farms, mining areas, and forests in rural areas contributes to persistent differences, most notably lower population densities (Gilford et al., 1981). By 1980, however, over two-thirds of the work force both inside and outside metropolitan areas was employed in three industries: service, manufacturing, and retail trade (U.S. Department of Commerce, Bureau of the Census, 1981).

The purpose of this chapter is to:

1. Describe the principal "rural" definitions applied by the federal government that affect health programs and policies, i.e., urban and rural areas (and populations) as defined by

the Bureau of the Census and metropolitan statistical areas as
defined by the Office of Management and Budget (OMB)
2. Describe the classifications used to distinguish different
   types of rural areas
3. Discuss how federal agencies have used these definitions to
   compile vital and health statistics and to implement programs
4. Discuss the strengths and weaknesses of rural definitions
   and classifications currently in use

Delineating "Rural" and "Urban" Areas

The concepts of "rural" and "urban" now exist as part of a
continuum. Although few would argue about the extremes of that
continuum—for example, an isolated farming community in
Texas at one extreme and New York City at the other—where to
draw the line between urban and rural has become more difficult.
Many federal policies, however, rely on dichotomous rural/urban
designations. This section describes the two most important dichotomous geographic designations: the Bureau of the Census's
urban and rural areas (and populations), and the OMB's metropolitan statistical areas and residual nonmetropolitan territory.
Several geographic classification schemes are then described that
portray the urban-rural continuum.

United States Bureau of the Census

According to the Census Bureau, urban and rural are "type-of-
area concepts rather than specific areas outlined on maps" (U.S.
Department of Commerce, Bureau of the Census, 1983a). The *urban
population* includes persons living in urbanized areas and those
living in places with 2,500 residents or more outside urbanized
areas. The population not classified as urban comprises the *rural
population*, that is, those living outside urbanized areas in "places"
with less than 2,500 residents and those living outside "places" in
the open countryside. Census-recognized "places" are either (1)
incorporated places such as cities, boroughs, towns, and villages;
or (2) closely settled population centers that are outside urbanized
areas, do not have corporate limits, and have a population of at

least 1,000. The rural population is divided further into farm and nonfarm populations.

Urbanized areas consist of a central core (a "central city or cities") and the contiguous, closely settled territory outside the city's political boundaries (the "urban fringe") that, combined, have a total population of at least 50,000 (U.S. Department of Commerce, Bureau of the Census, 1980). The boundary of an urbanized area is based primarily on a residential population density of at least 1,000 persons per square mile, although the area generally also includes less densely settled areas, such as industrial parks (U.S. Department of Commerce, Bureau of the Census, 1981). The boundaries of urbanized areas are not limited to preexisting county or state lines; rather they often follow the boundaries of small Census-defined geographic units such as census tracts and enumeration districts. Many urbanized areas cross county and/or state lines. The 1980 Census identified 373 urbanized areas in the United States and Puerto Rico (U.S. Department of Commerce, Bureau of the Census, 1985).

The Census definition of urban areas has changed considerably over time. Prior to 1900, the lower population limit for the size of places considered urban was set at either 4,000 or 8,000. The limit was lowered to 2,500 residents in 1900 (U.S. Department of Commerce, Bureau of the Census, 1975). This definition worked well until suburban development outside corporate boundaries became extensive. To improve the definition, people living in fairly densely populated areas (at least 1,000 persons per square mile) in the immediate vicinity of cities of 50,000 or more population were counted as urban instead of rural beginning in 1950 (Long and DeAre, 1982). With the exclusion of these suburban residents, the size of the 1950 rural population dropped from 62 million to 54 million (U.S. Department of Commerce, Bureau of the Census, 1975).

The *rural population* has been divided by the Census Bureau into the farm and nonfarm populations. The *farm population* includes people living in rural areas on properties of 1 acre of land or more where $1,000 or more of agricultural products were sold (or would have been sold) during the previous 12 months. In 1987, the farm population was estimated at 4,986,000, or about 8 percent of the rural population and 2 percent of the total resident U.S. population. In contrast, farm residents represented 30 percent of the population in 1920 (U.S. Department of Commerce, Bureau of the Census, 1988).

According to the 1980 Census, 73.7 percent of the U.S. population was urban, but the proportion ranged from a low of 33.8 percent in Vermont to 100 percent in the District of Columbia (U.S. Department of Commerce, Bureau of the Census, 1983b). Over 85 percent of the rural population lives in places or areas with fewer than 1,000 residents.

The Census Bureau's "urbanized" area concept does not apply to towns, cities, or population concentrations of less than 50,000. Those living nearby, but outside the limits of smaller cities or towns, are not counted as being part of an "urbanized" area, even though the "suburban" population may be large and economically integrated with the town. For example, the population surrounding the incorporated village of Hayward, Wisconsin (county seat of Sawyer County) exceeds the 1,456 population of Hayward. The residents of the surrounding area use Hayward's facilities, such as a nursing home and fire station, but are not included in the village population. This "undercount" has hampered the village's ability to obtain grants to improve area services (Gilford et al., 1981). Numerous areas such as Hayward that are considered "rural" by virtue of the fact that they are outside an urbanized area and have a population of 2,500 or less would be considered urban if the population immediately surrounding the corporate area were included. Many towns and villages have resolved this problem by annexing surrounding developed territory (Forstall, 1989).

The Office of Management and Budget: Metropolitan Statistical Areas

A *metropolitan statistical area* (MSA) is an economically and socially integrated geographic unit centered on a large urban area. In general terms, an MSA includes a large population center and adjacent communities that have a high degree of economic and social integration with that center (U.S. Department of Commerce, Bureau of the Census, 1988). This contrasts with the Census Bureau's *urban area,* which is defined solely on the basis of where people reside (i.e., population size and density). MSAs are defined by OMB and are used by federal agencies as the basis for collecting, tabulating, and publishing statistical data. Some federal agencies also use MSA designations to implement programs and allocate resources, although OMB does not define them with such applications in mind. The business community uses MSA data and rankings extensively, for example, in making investment decisions and assessing the desirability of markets (Schlosberg, 1989).

The official standards that are used to define MSAs are reviewed prior to each decennial Census. According to standards adopted for the 1980 Census, an MSA must have a city with 50,000 or more residents, or an urbanized area (as defined by the Census Bureau) with at least 50,000 people that is part of a county or counties that have at least 100,000 people. In most areas, counties are the building blocks of MSAs. In the six New England states, MSAs are composed of cities and towns, rather than whole counties.

MSAs often include more than one county. An MSA may be made up of one or more central counties containing the area's main population concentration and outlying counties that have close economic and social relationships with those central counties. To be included in the MSA, the outlying counties must have a specified level of commuting to the central counties and must also meet certain standards regarding metropolitan character, such as population density. Consolidated MSAs are large metropolitan complexes within which individual components are defined; these are in turn designated as primary MSAs.

Problems in MSA classification may occur when county boundaries do not conform closely to actual urban or suburban development. An MSA may inappropriately include nonsuburban areas located in the outlying sections of some counties. For example, in a spatially large county with a concentrated metropolitan area, a large, sparsely populated area may be included in the MSA. This problem occurs more frequently in the west, where counties are bigger than those in the east. On the other hand, an MSA may exclude suburban areas just across the county line. For example, a county with a suburban population that commutes to a neighboring MSA may be excluded from that MSA because it also includes a large, sparsely populated section and therefore has a low average population density. Although these problems occur, they occur infrequently (U.S. Department of Commerce, Office of Federal Statistical Policy and Standards, 1979, 1980).

About three-quarters (76.6 percent) of the U.S. population lived in the 275 MSAs designated as of 1983. These MSAs represent only 16.2 percent of the total U.S. land area (see fig. 2.1). Seventy-seven percent of U.S. counties (2,422 of 3,139 counties and county equivalents) are nonmetropolitan.

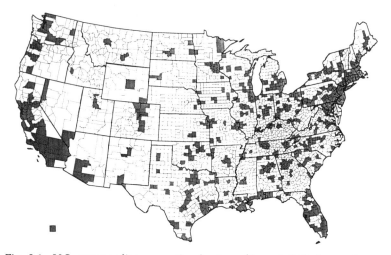

Fig. 2.1. U.S. metropolitan counties (metropolitan statistical areas), ac-
cording to 1986 U.S. Office of Management and Budget designation.
Source: Rural Health Research Program, University of North Carolina at
Chapel Hill. *Data source:* Area Resource File, Department of Health and
Human Services.

Before 1970, an MSA's "recognized large population nucleus"
had to include a central city with a population of at least 50,000 or
twin cities with a total population this large. Now there is no
minimum population size for an MSA's central city, and it is easier
to include contiguous populations in the urbanized area (Beale,
1984). With the relaxation of MSA criteria, some of the 58 MSAs
designated following the 1970 and 1980 Censuses are demographically dissimilar from those MSAs meeting earlier standards. For
example, of the 33 MSAs newly designated after the 1980 Census
that lacked a city of 50,000 or more residents, 25 had rural population percentages that were closer to nonmetropolitan norms (62
percent) than metropolitan norms (15 percent) (Beale, 1984). Furthermore, many of these do not have facilities and services traditionally associated with metropolitan areas, such as hospitals with
comprehensive services, a four-year college, a local bus service, a
television station, or a Sunday paper (Beale, 1984).

A few counties that have not qualified for MSA status on the
basis of demographic characteristics have become designated as
MSAs through the federal legislative process. Specifically, since

1983, one new MSA comprising two counties (Decatur, Alabama) has been created and the boundaries of two existing MSAs have been enlarged by statute (U.S. Executive Office of the President, Office of Management and Budget, 1983–1988). The proponents of the bill to create the Decatur, Alabama, MSA argued that "MSA status would encourage a measure of economic recovery to this area . . . without any additional financial burden on the Federal Government" (U.S. Congress, House of Representatives, 1988b). Hospitals located in the newly designated MSA of Decatur, Alabama, are expected to receive an additional $3 million per year in Medicare reimbursements because of this change from nonmetropolitan (rural) to metropolitan status. The increase in Medicare outlays for these two counties would, in aggregate, decrease reimbursement to other hospitals because the total amount of funding for the Medicare program was not changed by this act (U.S. Congress, House of Representatives, 1988a).

The MSA definition is designed strictly for statistical applications and not as a general-purpose geographic framework. In fact, according to official standards, "no Federal department or agency should adopt these statistical definitions for a nonstatistical program unless the agency head has determined that this is an appropriate use of the classification" (U.S. Department of Commerce, Office of Federal Statistical Policy and Standards, 1979, 1980). The OMB does not take into account or attempt to anticipate any nonstatistical uses that may be made of the MSA definitions and will not modify the definitions to meet the requirements of any nonstatistical program (U.S. Executive Office of the President, Office of Management and Budget, 1983–1988). Nonetheless, federal agencies often use MSA designations to implement their programs.

Relationship between Urban/Rural and Metropolitan/Nonmetropolitan Designations

Conceptually, the urban/rural and metropolitan/nonmetropolitan designations are quite different. Urban and rural are geographic designations based on population size and residential population densities, whereas the MSA concept embodies both a physical element (a city and its built-up suburbs) and a functional dimension (a more or less unified local labor market) (Long and

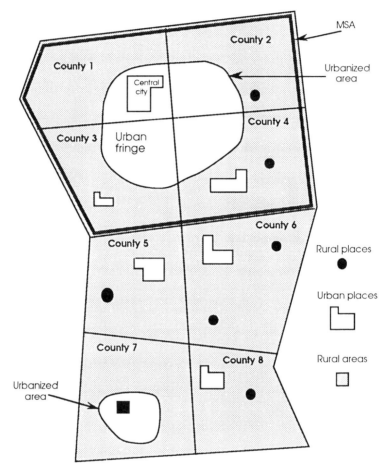

Fig. 2.2. Relationship among metropolitan statistical areas, urbanized areas, and urban and rural areas. Counties 1–4 comprise the MSA. *Urbanized areas* form the nucleus of the MSA and can span two or more counties (e.g., counties 1–4). There are a few urbanized areas in non-MSA counties (e.g., county 7). *Urban areas* include urbanized areas and places (e.g., cities and towns) with 2,500 or more residents. Such places are called *urban places*. *Rural places* are located outside urbanized areas and have fewer than 2,500 residents. *Rural areas* are the residential territory (shaded) left after urbanized areas and urban places are excluded. The MSA has rural areas within it.

Table 2.1. Population Inside and Outside MSAs by Urban and Rural Residence (1980)

	Population	Percent of MSA/non-MSA
U.S. total	226,545,805	
Inside MSAs	169,430,623	100.0
Urban	145,442,528	85.8
Urbanized areas	137,481,718	81.1
Central cities	66,222,207	39.1
Urban fringe	71,259,511	42.1
Rural	23,988,095	14.2
Outside MSAs	57,115,182	100.0
Urban	21,608,464	37.8
Rural	35,506,718	62.2

Source: U.S. Department of Commerce, Bureau of the Census (1981), table 6, pp. 1–39.

DeAre, 1982). The Census-defined urban population and the MSA population intersect but are by no means identical; they are even less congruent geographically. Common to both are residents of most urbanized areas, the densely settled areas that form the nuclei of the MSAs (see fig. 2.2). The Census's urban population includes the urbanized area population and those living outside urbanized areas in places with 2,500 or more residents. The MSA population generally includes all those living in the county or counties that contain the urbanized area and the residents of additional counties that are economically integrated with that metropolitan core. Forty percent of the 1980 rural population lived in MSAs, and 14 percent of the MSA population lived in rural areas (see table 2.1). About one-fourth of farm residents live in MSAs (U.S. Department of Commerce, Bureau of the Census, 1988).

The terms "rural area," "nonurbanized area," and "nonmetropolitan area" have all been used to display vital and health statistics or to implement federal policies in health and other areas. These "rural" definitions can be analyzed in terms of how well they include "rural areas" and how well they exclude "urban areas." The Census-defined "rural area" is the most specific measure, since it excludes urbanized areas and places with 2,500 residents or more. Thus, few would argue that an area designated as rural according to the Census definition is really urban. However, some might argue that the Census definition would incorrectly classify as urban small towns that are located far from a large population center. In contrast, the "nonurbanized area" definition includes as rural all territory outside of its densely populated area, regardless of population size. Thus, while all "rural areas" would be included, some cities and towns of as large as 40,000 residents would also be included, as well as some outer suburbs of large urban areas.

The non-MSA designation falls in between the other two designations. If non-MSAs are used to define rural areas, some large towns and cities located outside MSAs would be included as rural whereas small towns and sparsely populated areas within MSAs would be excluded from the rural category. This exclusion is less of a concern in the eastern United States, where counties are relatively small, and such towns would generally be expected to be relatively close to an urbanized area. However, in some of the large counties in the west, some areas within an MSA are far from an urbanized area.

Understanding Diversity within Rural Areas: Urban/Rural Typologies

Dichotomous measures of urbanity and rurality obscure not only important differences between urban and rural areas but also wide variations within rural areas. Consequently, there have been recommendations to implement a standard rural typology that would capture the elements of rural diversity and improve use and comparison of data (Hersh and Van Hook, 1989). In the absence of such standardized data, it is difficult to quantify rural health problems and to make informed policy decisions.

In this section, several county-based rural/urban typologies or classification schemes are described that incorporate one or more of the following measures:

- population size and density
- proximity to and relationship with urban areas
- degree of urbanization
- principal economic activity

Only county-based typologies are considered here, because the county is generally the smallest geographic unit for which data are available nationally. Counties also have several other characteristics that make them useful units of analysis: county boundaries are generally stable; counties can be aggregated up to the state level; and counties are important administrative units for health and other programs. For small-area analyses and for research purposes, zip codes may be useful units of analysis. However, zip code boundaries are not stable and sometimes cross county lines.

Typologies Used to Describe Nonmetropolitan Areas

Several typologies have been developed to classify nonmetropolitan counties. Nine county-based typologies are described in this section. These typologies are generally used for research purposes and have not yet been used by federal agencies to implement health policies or to present vital and health statistics. Before discussing specific typologies, four geographic/demographic measures common to most of the typologies are briefly described: (1) population size, (2) population density, (3) adjacency to metropolitan area, and (4) urbanization.

Population size. Population size may refer to the total population of the county or to the largest settlement in the county. Presentation of an area's population by settlement size helps to illustrate how the population is distributed. In 1980, 43 percent of the U.S. population lived in places with populations of less than 10,000 or the open countryside. The Census Bureau's urban definition depends in part on population size (i.e., those living in places of 2,500 or more outside of urbanized areas).

Population density. Population density is calculated by dividing the resident population of a geographic unit by its land area measured in square miles or square kilometers. In 1980, half of the U.S. population (excluding Alaska and Hawaii) lived in counties with less than 383 persons per square mile (Long and DeAre, 1982). Population density ranges from 64,395 persons per square mile in New York County, New York (Manhattan) to 0.1 person per square mile in Dillingham Census Division, Alaska. Urbanized areas are defined primarily by population density (i.e.,

territory with at least 1,000 residents per square mile). One draw-
back of population density is that it does not describe how the
population is distributed within an area. For example, a spatially
large county that includes both small, densely settled urban areas
and large, sparsely populated areas would have a population
density that masks such extremes.

Adjacency to metropolitan area. A county's adjacency to a metropolitan area can be measured geographically (e.g., sharing a boundary)
or functionally (e.g., proportion of residents commuting to an MSA
for work). Many residents of these adjacent counties, however, live
some distance from an urban center, particularly in large counties in
the West. Furthermore, natural geographic barriers or an absence of
roads may impede access to metropolitan areas.

Urbanization. Some typologies use various measures of the level
of urbanization to differentiate nonmetropolitan counties. Sometimes, urbanization is measured by the absolute or relative size of
the Census-defined urban population. For nonmetropolitan counties this generally means the population living in places with 2,500
or more residents or the proportion of the county's population
that is urban. In other typologies, an urbanized county is defined
by the size of the county's total population (e.g., counties with
25,000 or more residents).

Urbanization/Adjacency to Metropolitan Areas

Analysts at the U.S. Department of Agriculture (USDA) have
classified nonmetropolitan counties on two dimensions: (1) the
aggregate size of their urban population and (2) proximity/adja-
cency to metropolitan counties (see table 2.2) (McGranahan et al.,
1986). The urban population follows the Census Bureau's definition. Urbanized counties are distinguished from less urbanized
counties by the size of the urban population: urbanized counties
have at least 20,000 urban residents and less urbanized counties
have 2,500 to 19,999 urban residents. A nonmetropolitan county's
adjacency to an MSA is defined both by shared boundaries (i.e.,
touching an MSA at more than a single point) and by commuting
patterns (i.e., at least 1 percent of the county's labor force commutes to the central county or counties of the MSA). Nearly 40
percent of the nonmetropolitan counties are adjacent to MSAs,

Table 2.2. Classification of Nonmetropolitan Counties by Urbanization
and Proximity to Metropolitan Areas (1980)

Classification	Number of counties	Description
Urbanized adjacent	137	Counties with an urban population of at least 20,000 that are adjacent to a metropolitan county
Urbanized nonadjacent	151	Counties with an urban population of at least 20,000 that are not adjacent to a metropolitan county
Less-urbanized adjacent	552	Counties with an urban population of 2,500 to 19,999 that are adjacent to a metropolitan county
Less-urbanized nonadjacent	757	Counties with an urban population of 2,500 to 19,999 that are not adjacent to a metropolitan county
Rural adjacent	229	Counties that are completely rural or have fewer than 2,500 urban population that are adjacent to a metropolitan county
Rural nonadjacent	557	Counties that are completely rural or have fewer than 2,500 urban population that are not adjacent to a metropolitan county

Note: There were 2,383 nonmetropolitan counties as of 1980.
Sources: McGranahan et al. (1986); M. Butler (1991).

and just over half of the nonmetropolitan population resides in these adjacent counties.

This typology still masks differences among non-MSA counties. For example, both a county with one town of 20,000 and a county with eight towns of 2,500 would be considered urbanized under this typology. Yet the county with several small towns is unlikely to have the level of services of a county with its population concentrated into larger towns.

Adjacency to Metropolitan Areas/ Largest Settlement Size

Another county typology groups nonmetropolitan counties by adjacency to MSAs and by size of the largest settlement (see table 2.3) (Long and DeAre, 1982). Size of largest settlement is a useful parameter to include when analyzing health services, since large settlements are more likely to have hospitals and specialized health care providers. However, the presence of a large town or

Table 2.3. U.S. Population by County's Largest Settlement and
Adjacency to an MSA (1980)

	Population (1,000s)	Percent of U.S. population
U.S. total	226,505	100.0
Non-MSA counties	60,512	26.7
Counties not adjacent to an MSA		
Largest settlement		
Under 2,500	4,543	2.0
2,500 to 9,999	10,255	4.5
10,000 to 24,999	7,120	3.1
25,000 or more	4,124	1.8
Counties adjacent to an MSA		
Largest settlement		
Under 2,500	3,157	1.4
2,500 to 9,999	13,236	5.8
10,000 to 24,999	12,467	5.5
25,000 or more	5,610	2.5
MSA counties	165,994	73.3
Largest settlement		
Under 100,000	3,611	1.6
100,000 to 249,999	18,461	8.2
250,000 to 499,999	24,883	11.0
500,000 to 999,999	28,640	12.6
1,000,000 to 2,999,999	50,524	22.3
3,000,000 or more	39,875	17.6

Source: Adapted from Long and DeAre (1982).

city does not guarantee easy access to facilities for all residents of
a spatially large county.

Population Density: Incorporation of the Frontier Concept

The National Rural Health Association (NRHA) has proposed a
classification system that includes four types of rural areas (Patton, 1989):

- adjacent rural areas: counties contiguous to or within MSAs that are very similar to their rural neighbors
- urbanized rural areas: counties with 25,000 or more residents but distant from an MSA
- frontier areas: counties with population densities of less than 6 persons per square mile, which are the most remote areas
- countryside rural areas: the remainder of the country not covered by other rural designations

This typology includes some important concepts not covered by other typologies, such as the concept of the "frontier" area. This typology also differs from other typologies because it includes some counties within MSAs (i.e., in the adjacent rural area category). Since the categories are not mutually exclusive, however, some counties will fall into more than one group. For example, under this typology three of fourteen counties in Arizona (Apache, Coconino, and Mohave) would be both "urbanized rural areas" and "frontier areas" because the counties' populations exceed 25,000 residents and the population density is less than six persons per square mile. County population size is a poor indicator in the west because many counties there are much larger than elsewhere.

Urbanization/Population Density

Two other rural typologies incorporate population density and urbanization. The first is a classification developed by Bluestone and the second is a modification by Clifton of that classification (see table 2.4). Urbanization is defined in terms of the proportion of the county that is urban (i.e., lives in towns of 2,500 or more). An advantage of using the percent of a county's population that is urban is that this indicator is not influenced much by the size of the county, or by a county's including a large stretch of unpopulated territory. Density is heavily affected by these conditions. Combining measures of urbanization and density provides some indication of the degree of population concentration or dispersion. However, as with the USDA typology, a county with one town of 20,000 and a county with eight towns of 2,500 may not be distinguished under this scheme.

Table 2.4. Bluestone and Clifton County Classifications Based on
Urbanization and Population Density

	Percent urban	Population per square mile
Bluestone classification		
Metropolitan	>85	>100
		or
	>50	>500
Urban	<85	100–500
Semiisolated urban	>50	<100
Densely settled rural	<50	50–100
Sparsely settled rural with some urban population	<50	<50
Sparsely settled rural with no urban population	0	<50
Clifton classification		
Urban	50	200
Semiurban	50	30–200
Densely settled rural	<50	>30
Rural	<100	<30

Source: Sinclair and Manderscheid (1974).

Distance from an MSA or Population Center

Two rural indexes are based on distance from an MSA or population center. These rural indexes are different from typologies in
that they are continuous (e.g., a scale from 1 to 100) rather than
categorical measures. Hathaway et al. developed a size-distance
index that includes two measures: miles from an MSA and the
population of that MSA (Sinclair and Manderscheid, 1974). Smith
and Parvin considered three county characteristics in their rural
index: population-proximity, population density, and employment in agriculture, forestry, or fisheries (Smith and Parvin, 1973;
U.S. Congress, House of Representatives, 1983).

A county's population-proximity indicates the relative access to
adjacent counties' populations. Population-proximity is measured
as the county population plus the size-distance ratio of surround-

ing counties. The population-proximity is "the sum of the total population in the reference county and the sum of the ratios of the number of persons in all counties within 125 miles of the reference county divided by the distance in miles between the county seat in the reference county and the county seat in each county within the specified distance" (U.S. Congress, House of Representatives, 1983). The combination in a typology of distance to adjacent population centers and size of those populations is attractive because distance is a good access indicator and population size indicates service availability. The typologies incorporating these measures may be most informative for geographically small counties. For large counties, however, the distance from one county seat to the next is unlikely to be applicable to those living at a distance from the county seat.

Commuting-Employment Patterns

A relatively new county classification system incorporates measures of population size, urbanization, commuting patterns of workers, and the relationships between workplace and place of residence (Pickard, 1988). The classification criteria are shown in table 2.5. The inclusion of employment and commuting measures may allow this typology to identify groups of counties that are economically related, such as service and labor market areas.

Economic and Sociodemographic Characteristics

Nonmetropolitan counties have also been classified according to their major economic bases, land uses, or population characteristics (see table 2.5) (Bender et al., 1985). Fifteen percent of nonmetropolitan counties (370 of 2,443 counties in the 48 conterminous states) remain unclassified using this approach. Among the counties that are classified, 70 percent fall into only one of the seven categories; the remaining 30 percent fall into two or more categories (Ross, 1986).

Some of the data used to develop this classification, such as farm employment, are now a decade old, and it is likely that given the continued diversification of the rural economy since the late 1970s, even fewer counties would be classified into one of these groups today. On the other hand, many rural economies remain small and dependent on a single industry or occupation despite the economic diversification (Bender et al., 1985).

Table 2.5. Classification of Nonmetropolitan Counties by Economic and Sociodemographic Characteristics

Farming-dependent counties	702 counties concentrated largely in the plains portion of the north central region. Farming contributed a weighted annual average of 20 percent or more of total labor and proprietor income over the five years from 1975 to 1979.
Manufacturing-dependent counties	678 counties concentrated in the southeast. Manufacturing contributed 30 percent or more of total labor and proprietor income in 1979.
Mining-dependent counties	200 counties concentrated in the west and in Appalachia. Mining contributed 20 percent or more of total labor and proprietor income in 1979.
Specialized government counties	315 counties scattered throughout the country. Government activities contributed 25 percent or more of total labor and proprietor income in 1979.
Persistent poverty counties	242 counties concentrated in the South, especially along the Mississippi Delta and in parts of Appalachia. Per capita family income in the county was in the lowest quintile in each of the years 1950, 1959, 1969, and 1979.
Federal lands counties	247 counties concentrated in the west. Federal land was 33 percent or more of the land area in a county in 1977.
Destination retirement counties	515 counties concentrated in several northern lake states as well as in the south and southwest. For the 1970 to 1980 period, net immigration rates of people aged 60 and over were 15 percent or more of the expected 1980 population aged 60 and over. Retirement counties are disproportionately affected by entitlement programs benefiting the aged.

Note: The number of nonmetropolitan counties does not add up to the total number (2,443) because the categories are not mutually exclusive and 370 counties do not fit any of the categories.
Source: Bender et al. (1985).

Conclusion

In summary, several typologies for describing nonmetropolitan counties have been developed, incorporating measures of population size and density, urbanization, adjacency and relationship to MSAs, and principal economic activity (see table 2.6). Although it

Table 2.6. Features of the Nine County-based Typologies

Typology	Measures					
	Population size	Density	Urbani- zation	Adjacency	Distance	Economy
USDA-1 (McGranahan et al., 1986)	—	—	✓	✓	—	—
Long and DeAre (1982)	✓	—	—	✓	—	—
National Rural Health Association (cited in Patton, 1989)	✓	✓	—	✓	—	—
Bluestone (cited in Sinclair and Manderscheid, 1974)	—	✓	✓	—	—	—
Clifton (cited in Sinclair and Manderscheid, 1974)	—	✓	✓	—	—	—
Parvin and Smith (cited in U.S Congress, House of Representatives, 1983)	✓	—	—	—	✓	—
Hathaway (cited in Sinclair and Manderscheid, 1974)	✓	—	—	—	✓	—
Pickard (1988)	✓	—	✓	—	—	✓
USDA-2 (Bender et al., 1985)	—	—	—	—	—	✓

Source: Office of Technology Assessment, U.S. Congress (1989).

is desirable to have a standardized typology to portray the diversity of rural areas, the potential uses of typologies are varied and thus require the inclusion of different measures. For example, to study the geographic variation of access to health care, a typology that includes population size, density, and distance to large settlements is of interest. To study health personnel labor market areas, however, a typology based on economic areas, market areas, or worker commuting patterns is preferable. On the other hand, rural economists or sociologists may be more interested in identifying counties with economies dependent on farming, mining, or forestry.

Although no one typology meets all potential needs, there are several desirable features of any typology. For example, for many purposes it is helpful to have typologies with mutually exclusive (i.e., nonoverlapping) categories. The NRHA's typology includes frontier (less than six persons per square mile) and urbanized rural counties (population of 25,000 or more and not adjacent to an MSA). Yet it is possible for counties to meet both criteria.

The concept of urbanization is incorporated into several of the typologies. In some cases, urbanization is determined by the absolute or relative size of a county's urban population and, in others, by the size of a county's largest settlement. When the size of the urban population is used, a county with one large city with the balance of the county sparsely populated would be indistinguishable from a county with several smaller towns. As levels of resources are likely to be city size–dependent, typologies using this measure of urbanization may not discriminate well for some applications. On the other hand, although largest settlement size might be indicative of level of services available in the county, it is not informative of how remote those services might be for some county residents. In geographically small counties, large settlements are likely to be accessible to all county residents. In the west, however, counties may be as large as some eastern states, and some measure of proximity would be useful to indicate physical access. Measures of how evenly the population is distributed might also be useful for large counties.

The Hoover index is a measure of population concentration or dispersion. The index ranges from zero, which indicates a perfectly uniform distribution in which each subarea has the same proportion of total population as it does of land area, to 100, which represents the concentration of all the population into a single subarea (Long and DeAre, 1982). To estimate county population dispersion, subcounty geographic areas would be used. Other methods to measure population concentration or dispersion include the nearest-neighbor statistic or the quadrat technique, but both require a geographic information system incorporating longitude and latitude measures (Dahmann, 1989; Joseph and Phillips, 1984; Meade et al., 1988). Several of the typologies incorporate an adjacent-to-MSA measure, which is an indicator of access to level of services. The proportion of a county's population that is urban is a useful measure in large western counties because, unlike population density, it is a measure that is not influenced much by size of county or by population distribution.

Nonmetropolitan county data can also be disaggregated regionally by state or groups of states (e.g., the four Census regions or nine Census divisions), or by economic areas (e.g., Bureau of Economic Analysis Areas). The Bureau of the Census defines "county groups" that are usually contiguous counties that combined have a population of 100,000 or more. These counties are generally grouped according to meaningful state regions such as planning districts (U.S. Department of Commerce, Bureau of the Census, 1983a).

A new category of nonmetropolitan area called "micropolitan area" has recently been described (Thomas, 1989). Although not a typology, the new category does distinguish nonmetropolitan areas that exert social and economic influences on their regions similar to those exerted by metropolitan areas on a larger scale. Most micropolitan areas are single counties but a few span two counties or are independent cities. Micropolitan counties are relatively large (40,000 or more residents) and include a central "core city" with at least 15,000 residents. Many micropolitan areas are college towns, sites of military bases, and retirement areas. More than 15 million people or about one-quarter of nonmetropolitan residents live in the 219 identified micropolitan areas.

The Availability of Vital and Health Statistics for Nonmetropolitan Areas

Given the diversity of nonmetropolitan areas, it is important to present vital and health statistics by state, region, or nonmetropolitan typology. Data from the decennial Census and national vital statistics (e.g., natality and mortality data) are published for nonmetropolitan areas by state and degree of urbanization, but few other sources of health information are published along these dimensions. For example, the National Center for Health Statistics does not publish detailed nonmetropolitan data (e.g., cross-tabulated by federal region) in their reports on National Health Interview and National Medical Care Utilization and Expenditure Surveys. Sometimes, limitations of the way in which the data are collected, such as the sample size or frame, limit the extent to

Table 2.7. Proportion of the Population Sixty-five Years Old and Older by Metropolitan/Nonmetropolitan and Urban/Rural Residence

Area	U.S. population	Percent age 65 and over
Metropolitan	169,430,577	10.7
Nonmetropolitan	57,115,228	13.0
Urban	167,054,638	11.4
Rural	59,491,167	10.9
Metropolitan		
Urban	145,451,315	10.9
Central cities	67,854,918	11.8
Not central cities	77,596,397	10.2
Rural	23,979,262	9.0
Nonmetropolitan		
Urban	21,603,323	14.3
Rural	35,511,905	12.2

Source: U.S. Department of Commerce, Bureau of the Census (1981).

which nonmetropolitan data can be displayed. In general, however, survey data files are available for public use and can be analyzed by area.

The choice of the definition of "rural" used to present demographic and health data can make a substantive difference. For example, whether a disproportionate number of rural residents are elderly depends on how rural is defined (see table 2.7). The elderly appear to make up a larger proportion of the total population in nonmetropolitan than metropolitan areas (13.0 versus 10.7 percent). Using the urban/rural categories, however, the opposite is true—there is a greater proportion of elderly residents in urban than rural areas (11.4 versus 10.9). The explanation for this discrepancy appears to be that there are proportionately more persons 65 and older living in urban nonmetropolitan areas (14.3 percent) and fewer in rural metropolitan areas (9.0 percent). Moreover, when nonmetropolitan county MSA-adjacency and size of the urbanized population are considered, the aged appear to be overrepresented in the less urbanized and nonadjacent counties.

Infant mortality is also better understood by looking beyond metropolitan/nonmetropolitan comparisons. The U.S. Department of Health and Human Services (DHHS) publishes data on infant mortality for urban and "not urban" places within metropolitan and nonmetropolitan counties (nonmetropolitan urban places are defined as those with populations of 10,000 or more). Within U.S. nonmetropolitan areas (1985–1986), white infant mortality rates were lower in nonurban places than in urban places (9.3 versus 9.9). Black infant mortality, in contrast, is higher in nonurban places (17.8 versus 16.5). In some nonmetropolitan areas, like Alabama, infant mortality is higher in the more rural areas for both whites and blacks.

In summary, quite different conclusions about the rural population may be reached by changing the definition of rural areas. Furthermore, important within-area variations are obscured when national data are not published for sub-nonmetropolitan areas.

The problem of limited rural data is not a new one for policymakers. In 1981, the National Academy of Sciences addressed the issue in a report, *Rural America in Passage: Statistics for Policy*. A panel on Statistics for Rural Development Policy composed of agricultural economists, statisticians, geographers, sociologists, and demographers made a number of recommendations for improving the perceived poor availability and quality of rural statistical data bases. The panel recommended that the federal government "take a more active role in the coordination of statistical activities and in developing and promulgating common definitions and other statistical standards that are appropriate for implementation at the Federal, State, and local levels." The panel concluded that a single definition of "rural" is neither feasible nor desirable but recommended that data be organized in a building-block approach so that different definitions and typologies could be constructed. The panel recognized the need for a common aggregation scheme for counties. It recommended the development of a standard classification of nonmetropolitan counties related to the level of urbanization. The panel recommended that, if possible, the county classification should be supplemented by a distinction between urban and rural areas within counties (Gilford et al., 1981).

The lack of consistent county coding poses difficulties for those interested in developing county-based definitions and typologies. Unique county identifiers called county Federal Information Processing Standards codes are provided by the National Institute of Measurement and Technology but are not universally used (Bonnen, 1988). The panel recommended that federal and state data be recorded with such county codes to permit tabulations for individual counties and groups of counties. Adherence to a county coding system would facilitate aggregation of information regardless of how rural is defined. However, since the report was issued in 1981, few of its recommendations have been implemented (Bonnen, 1988).

The relative merits of the county-based typologies for health service planning and research can be evaluated using the Area Resource File (ARF), a county-level data base maintained by the Health Resources and Services Administration (U.S. Department of Health and Human Services, Public Health Service, 1988). The file contains data necessary for the Bureau of Health Professions to carry out its mandated program of research and analysis of the geographic distribution and supply of health personnel. Population, economic, and mortality data, and measures of health personnel, health education, and hospital resources, are included in the file (U.S. Department of Health and Human Services, Public Health Service, 1988).

The ARF has been used to show how the availability of physician and hospital resources varies by type of nonmetropolitan area (Kindig et al., 1988). For example, when physician availability is examined by type of county, wide variations in physician-to-population ratios are evident. The average physician-to-population ratio is 64 per 100,000 in nonmetropolitan counties, but it ranges from 131 per 100,000 in high-density counties to a low of 45 per 100,000 in persistent poverty counties. Somewhat surprisingly, there appear to be relatively more physicians in non-adjacent than adjacent nonmetropolitan counties (67 compared to 59 per 100,000). A possible explanation is that physicians serving many of the residents of the adjacent nonmetropolitan counties are preferentially locating in the outlying suburban areas of MSAs.

Maps effectively illustrate geographic variation in health status and access to health care resources. U.S. cancer atlases have been published at the county level, providing a visualization of geographic patterns of cancer mortality not apparent from tabular data (U.S. Department of Health and Human Services, Public Health Service, 1987). For example, rural women in the lower socioeconomic classes have high rates of cervical cancer and, for white women, maps show concentrations of cervical cancer throughout the south, especially in Appalachia.

Maps of the United States by county show higher death rates owing to unintentional injury (e.g., house fires and drownings) and motor vehicle crashes in rural areas, particularly in western, sparsely populated counties. The large volume of travel on major routes traversing rural areas does not account for the high rural death rates. Instead, road characteristics, travel speeds, seatbelt use, types of vehicles, and availability of emergency care are factors that may contribute to the excess of motor vehicle crash deaths in rural areas (Baker et al., 1987).

Using OMB and Census Designations to Implement Health Programs

There is no uniformity in how rural areas are defined for purposes of federal program administration and distribution of funds. Even within agencies different definitions may be used. This may occur when agencies implement programs or policies for which rural areas have been defined legislatively. For example, the MSA/non-MSA designations are used to categorize hospitals as located in urban or rural areas for purposes of hospital reimbursement under Medicare. On the other hand, in the case of clinics certified under the Rural Health Clinics Act, "rural" is defined as Census Bureau–designated nonurbanized areas. Certified clinics receive cost-based reimbursement from Medicare and Medicaid.

The Rural Health Clinics Act

Ambulatory services can be reimbursed on an at-cost basis by Medicare and Medicaid if facilities and providers meet certification requirements of the Rural Health Clinics Act (P.L. 95-210). To be certified, a practice must be located in a rural area that is designated either as a health manpower shortage area (HMSA) or a medically underserved area (MUA). The practice must use a midlevel practitioner (physician assistant or nurse practitioner) at least 60 percent of the time that the practice is open. There has been renewed interest in this act following an increase in the ceiling of reasonable costs reimbursed by Medicare and Medicaid programs. The payment cap is indexed to the Medicare Economic Index (Rosenberg, 1988).

Rural areas, for purposes of the Rural Health Clinics Act, are "areas not delineated as urbanized areas in the last census conducted by the Census Bureau." Nonurbanized areas encompass a larger area than either the non-MSA or the Census-defined rural areas. Therefore, rural health clinics can be located within an MSA or in a non-MSA town with a population of 2,500 or more (such a town is urban according to the Census Bureau).

In summary, for purposes of hospital reimbursement under Medicare, the MSA designation is used (with certain specific exceptions) to distinguish urban from rural hospitals. Persistent MSA/non-MSA hospital cost differences have been noted since the prospective payment system (PPS) rates were first established, but it is likely that MSA location is an indirect measure of hospital cost. Hospital-specific measures are being sought to replace the MSA adjustment in the PPS formula.

Although the Health Care Financing Administration (HCFA) has chosen not to use urbanized areas to refine labor market areas, HCFA does use urbanized area designations when certifying hospitals and clinics under the Rural Health Clinics Act. Rural health clinics must be located in nonurbanized areas that are designated as either an HMSA or an MUA. This liberal interpretation of "rural" (e.g., it includes some areas within MSAs) seems appropriate, given the requirement that the area must also be medically underserved. This allows some medically underserved areas within MSAs—but isolated from an urbanized area by factors other than distance—to be certified.

Providing Services in "Frontier" Areas

Health services may be difficult to provide in large, sparsely populated areas. Areas with a population density of six persons per square mile or fewer, called "frontier" areas, are common west of the Mississippi river (Popper, 1986). In 1980, by this definition, there were at least 378 frontier counties with a total population of nearly 3 million persons (Stambler, 1989). It may take an hour or more for residents of frontier areas to reach health providers and facilities. Frontier physicians tend to be generalists, solely responsible for a large service area, and have limited access to hospitals and health care technology (Elison, 1986). Recognizing the unique characteristics of frontier areas, the DHHS in early 1986 agreed to use different criteria to evaluate Community Health Center (CHC) grantees (and new applicants for CHC support) and National Health Service Corps sites. Frontier areas were defined as

> Those areas located throughout the country which are character-
> ized by a small population base (generally 6 persons per square
> mile or fewer) which is spread over a considerable geographic area.
> (U.S. Department of Health and Human Services, 1986)

To be eligible for Bureau of Health Care Delivery and Assistance
support as a frontier area, the following service area criteria must
be met:

> *Service Area:* a rational area in the frontier will have at least 500
> residents within a 25-mile radius of the health services delivery site
> or within the rationally established trade area. Most areas will have
> between 500 to 3,000 residents and cover large geographic areas.
> *Population Density:* the service area will have six or fewer persons
> per square mile.
> *Distance:* the service area will be such that the distance from a
> primary care delivery site within the service area to the next level of
> care will be more than 45 miles and/or the average travel time more
> than 60 minutes. When defining the "next level of care," we are refer-
> ring to a facility with 24-hour emergency care, with 24-hour capability
> to handle an emergency caesarean section or a patient having a heart
> attack and some specialty mix to include at a minimum, obstetric,
> pediatric, internal medicine, and anesthesia services.
> (U.S. Department of Health and Human Services, 1986)

Some state health departments have had trouble identifying
service areas meeting these criteria (New Mexico State Health and
Environment Department, 1987). Whole counties can be identified
as frontier areas on the basis of population density, but available
subcounty geographic units are sometimes inadequate for identifying health service areas. Population data from the 1980 Census
are available for subcounty areas such as Census County Divisions and Enumeration Districts, but these areas may be large and
may not represent a rational health service area. Some states (e.g.,
New York) have defined primary care service areas. Zip codes
may be aggregated to form a rational service area, but this poses
some technical difficulties (Licht, 1989). Some investigators have
used zip code–level census data to describe three types of rural
area based upon density within zip code: semirural (density of
sixteen to thirty persons per square mile); rural (density of six to
fifteen persons per square mile); and frontier (density of less than
six persons per square mile) (De la Torre et al., 1987). Following
the 1990 Census, Block Numbering Areas will be available for all
nonurbanized areas.

It is useful to distinguish frontier area counties with evenly distributed small settlements from counties with one or two large population settlements and large areas with little or no settlement. For example, the health service needs of two frontier counties in New Mexico with similar population densities differ because of the way the populations are distributed. One county has a total population of approximately 8,000, of whom about 6,000 live in one town. In contrast, the other county has a total population of 2,500 living in six widely dispersed towns. If suitable subcounty areas were available, the Hoover Index, which measures population concentration or dispersion, could be used to distinguish between these counties. An automated geographic information system called TIGER (Topologically Integrated Geographic Encoding and Referencing system) has been developed that will enhance the ability to conduct spatial analyses of population data from the 1990 decennial Census (McKenzie and LaMacchia, 1987). TIGER has been developed jointly by the U.S. Geological Survey and the U.S. Bureau of the Census.

Conclusions

The concepts of "rural" and "urban" exist as part of a continuum, but federal policies generally rely on dichotomous urban/rural differences based on designations of the OMB or the Bureau of the Census. OMB's MSA designation includes a large population center and adjacent counties that have a high degree of economic and social integration with that center. The Census Bureau's urban areas include densely settled "urbanized areas" plus places with populations of 2,500 or more outside urbanized areas. "Rural" areas are designated by exclusion: they are those areas not classified as either MSA or urban. About one-quarter of the U.S. population resides in non-MSAs and rural areas. The identified populations are different but overlapping. Forty percent of the population identified as rural in the 1980 Census lived in MSAs, and 14 percent of the MSA population lived in rural areas.

One may analyze how well such "rural" definitions as "nonmetropolitan area," "rural area," and "nonurbanized area" include "rural areas" and how well they exclude "urban areas." For example, we intuitively associate farming with "rural," but about one-fourth of farm residents live in MSAs (U.S. Department of

Commerce, Bureau of the Census, 1988). Some might argue that isolated towns with just over 2,500 residents are inappropriately excluded from the Census Bureau's rural definition. Others may argue that, when non-MSAs are defined as rural, over 100 towns with populations of 25,000 or more are inappropriately included. Moreover, when MSAs are used to define "urban" in spatially large counties, small towns that are far from an urbanized area are inappropriately called urban.

Dichotomous measures of urbanity and rurality mask key distinctions between urban and rural areas as well as wide variations within particular rural areas. Thus it has been suggested that a standard rural typology reflective of the elements of rural diversity be implemented to help improve use and comparison of data. This chapter has reviewed nine county-based rural/urban typologies or classification schemes that incorporate one or more of the following measures: population size and density; proximity to and relationship with urban areas; degree of urbanization; and principal economic activity. Although a standard typology may seem desirable, it will be difficult to arrive at, because the different typologies are designed and have merit for various purposes, some of which conflict.

For purposes of health services planning and research, a typology based on largest settlement size is useful, because the level of available health resources is likely to be related to the size of a city. In spatially small counties, large settlements are likely to be quite accessible to all county residents. In the west, however, counties can be several times as large as in the east, and some measure of proximity would be useful. A measure of population concentration and dispersion, or distance to a large settlement, could serve as an indicator of access to those services. Of the typologies reviewed in this chapter, the one likely to measure best both level of and access to services is a typology that incorporates a county's largest settlement and the county's adjacency to an MSA. Other typologies that categorize counties according to employment and commuting patterns could be used to refine the definition of labor market areas, an important component of the Medicare PPS formula (U.S. Department of Health and Human Services, 1989).

Rural areas are not defined uniformly for purposes of federal program administration or distribution of funds. Different designations may, in fact, be used by the same agency. For example, Congress has directed the HCFA to use OMB's MSA designations to categorize hospitals as urban or rural for purposes of hospital reimbursement under Medicare, but to use the Census Bureau's nonurbanized area designation to certify health facilities under the Rural Health Clinics Act.

The relative merits of county-based typologies for particular applications can be evaluated by using the ARF, a county-level data base maintained by the Health Resources and Services Administration. In addition, visual aids such as maps can effectively serve as an analytic device to illustrate geographic variation in health status and access to health care resources and could further the development and evaluation of typologies. In the spatially large western counties, subcounty geographic units need to be employed to help identify health service areas with special characteristics, such as those that are "frontier" (i.e., have six or fewer persons per square mile).

The choice of definition for "rural" that is used to present demographic and health data can make a substantive difference. For example, whether a disproportionate number of rural residents are elderly depends on how rural is defined. Furthermore, wide variations in health status indicators within nonmetropolitan areas will not be apparent unless nonmetropolitan data are disaggregated by region, urbanization, proximity to urban areas, or other relevant factors.

Chapter 3

Death Rates in Rural America 1939–1981
Convergence and Poverty

DONA SCHNEIDER AND
MICHAEL R. GREENBERG

Now, knowing that the average length of the life of mankind in towns has been much less than in the country, and that the average amount of disease and misery and of vice and crime has been much greater in towns, this would be a very dark prospect for civilization, if it were not that modern Science has beyond all question determined many of the causes of the special evils by which men are afflicted in towns, and placed means in our hands for guarding against them.

Frederick Law Olmsted (1822–1903),
Public Parks and the Enlightenment of Towns [1970]

However, the industrial revolution is not just history—it is still present. Those were the days of domestic pollution, these are the days of industrial pollution, for we are now grappling with the problems of safely controlling and disposing of the materials which spill out of and are thrown away by factories, foundries, refineries, and all the other elements of an industrial nation. . . .
Those at most disadvantage from these various potentially harmful environmental factors tend to be the relatively unskilled, or the manual or industrial workers and their families, living in areas of considerable industrial development, with all its associated problems. . . .

Anthony J. Rowland and Paul Cooper,
Environment and Health (1983)

And so, the myth continues: urban places remain degraded and unhealthy while people living in rural areas enjoy clean air, pure water, and better health. Although this may have been so earlier in this century, urbanization is no longer a synonym for high mortality rates, and rural living no longer automatically means healthy living. In this chapter we examine the relationship of U.S. death rates over forty years for whites thirty-five to sixty-four years old to changes in states' levels of both urbanization and poverty, using rank correlations and rate ratios. We argue that poverty is a new key to understanding health outcomes and that rural poverty, in particular, now is obvious in U.S. mortality trends.

Convergence and Poverty as Explanations of Mortality Trends

Regional death rates in the United States are converging toward the national rate for many causes of death, but not all (Greenberg, 1987a). For most cancers, heart diseases, and diabetes, convergence of rates between urban states like New York or New Jersey and rural states like Mississippi or West Virginia has been demonstrated for both white males and white females. This narrowing of rates is partially explained by better diagnosis and reporting systems for cancer in rural areas. High rates of interregional migration also partially explain some of this rate convergence. The most plausible explanation for the convergence of cancer mortality rates, however, is the increasing homogeneity of lifestyles across the nation, especially in smoking, drinking, and nutritional habits (Greenberg, 1983; Calkins, 1987).

For other causes of death, convergence of rates is not always demonstrable. For instance, a study of death rates from suicide, homicide and accidents among young white Americans from the 1940s to the 1980s showed geographic stability, not rate convergence. Six western mountain states (Arizona, Idaho, Montana, Nevada, New Mexico, and Wyoming) maintained rates 30 to 60 percent higher than the national rate for the entire forty-year period, and four northeastern states (Connecticut, Massachusetts, New Jersey and Rhode Island) maintained the lowest rates (Greenberg et al., 1985). In yet other instances—that of white female lung cancer, for example—urban/rural differences in mortality rates are actually increasing, not decreasing (Greenberg et al., 1983).

The geographic pattern of death in the United States, then, cannot be expressed as a single trend. It reflects many trends, depending upon the specific cause of death. Convergence of death rates—once commonly associated with urbanization and caused by increasing homogeneity of culture, population migration, and other factors—offers one explanation for these trends, but it does not explain the entire picture. We suggest that the localization of poverty in some regions and the localization of wealth in others is a second major force at work influencing these rates. To test this hypothesis, we review the major causes of death in the United States for the period 1939–1981 and relate the resultant patterns to two explanations—urbanization, the old standard explanation, and poverty.

Testing the Explanations

Hypotheses concerning urbanization and poverty as competing forces were tested, using state mortality data for major causes of death for the years 1939–1981. Using *Vital Statistics of the United States* for mortality counts and the U.S. Bureau of the Census for population-at-risk estimates, we calculated age-adjusted death rates for nine major causes of death for white males and white females for each of the forty-eight continental United States for the three-year time period surrounding each Census year, 1940–1980. In other words, we calculated age-adjusted death rates for 1939–1941, 1949–1951, 1959–1961, 1969–1971, and 1979–1981. We used white data only for the thirty-five to sixty-four-year-old age group and used the U.S. population for the Census year 1960 as the population standard. White data and thirty-five to sixty-four-year-olds were chosen because, as a group, they are a more sensitive barometer of premature death than is the total population since they exclude the elderly, minorities, those deaths resulting from infant mortality, and the violent deaths of young adults, including casualties of war.

We reviewed nine major causes of death at the state level: infectious diseases, diabetes, heart diseases, suicide, homicide, accidents, cancers, cerebrovascular diseases, and all other causes. These categories reflect the major, chronic, and violent causes of death for our age cohort. The age-adjusted rates for each state were ranked for each cause of death for each of the five time periods, with the highest rate being assigned rank one. We then ranked the states for percent urban (the surrogate for rural) as defined by the U.S. Bureau of the Census–persons living in incorporated places of 2,500 inhabitants or more and in other areas classified as urban under special rules relating to population size and density. Finally, we ranked each state by per capita personal income (the surrogate for poverty) for each time period using data from the *Statistical Abstract of the United States*. The state with the lowest percent urban (highest percent rural) and the lowest per capita personal income (highest poverty level) were ranked first. Low rankings, then, determined which states were poorest and most rural during the time periods specified. Conversely, high rankings denoted more urbanization and more personal wealth.

Mortality Trends in the United States

Before examining the changing relationships among mortality, urbanization, and poverty, we briefly examine national trends in mortality in the thirty-five to sixty-four-year-old age group. A review of age-adjusted mortality rates shows that American death rates have been decreasing over the past several decades. For instance, overall mortality for white males thirty-five to sixty-four years old was 1,243.5 per 100,000 in 1939–1941. By 1979–1981 that figure had dropped to 770.7. Pronounced decreases in rates for white males occurred for deaths from influenza/pneumonia (59.4 to 9.0), diabetes (22.2 to 10.4), heart diseases (397.2 to 303.6), suicide (40.5 to 22.7), accidents (114.2 to 53.8), and cerebrovascular diseases (78.6 to 26.7) over that forty-year period. Only homicide (7.8 to 10.9) and cancer (148.5 to 199.5) increased for middle-aged white males between 1939–1941 and 1979–1981.

For white middle-aged females the downward trends in mortality cover all but one category of death. Overall mortality decreased from 827.4 in 1939–1941 to 398.8 in 1979–1981. Rates fell for influenza/pneumonia (35.5 to 4.7), diabetes (38.7 to 8.6), heart diseases (186.9 to 92.9), suicide (12.6 to 9.3), accidents (28.4 to 17.8), cancer (194.4 to 162.9), and cerebrovascular diseases (74.7 to 21.5). Only homicide showed a rate increase, from 1.7 to 2.9.

Although the American death rate decreased between 1939–1941 and 1979–1981, regional differences in mortality rates remained apparent. Not all states or regions had the same downward mortality trends by cause that the United States as a whole exhibited. In order to determine whether these patterns could be explained by a correlation between age-adjusted mortal-

Table 3.1. Spearman Rank Correlations Relating Age-Adjusted Death Rates for Whites to Percent Urban (1939–1941, 1959–1961, and 1979–1981)

	White males			White females		
	1939–1941	1959–1961	1979–1981	1939–1941	1959–1961	1979–1981
All causes	-0.40*	-0.10	0.32*	-0.46*	-0.55*	-0.04
Influenza/pneumonia	0.11	-0.30*	-0.11	0.50*	-0.30*	0.27*
Diabetes	-0.53*	-0.28*	-0.08	-0.61*	-0.38*	-0.19
Heart diseases	-0.63*	-0.25*	0.38*	-0.66*	-0.45*	0.15
Suicide	-0.28*	0.30*	0.29*	-0.59*	-0.25*	0.15
Homicide	0.49*	0.15	0.19	0.13	0.05	-0.02
Accidents	0.11	0.50*	0.54*	-0.27*	0.18	0.19
Cancer	-0.88*	-0.46*	0.32*	-0.78*	-0.47*	-0.15
Cerebrovascular diseases	0.12	0.30*	0.48*	0.08	0.13	0.31*
Other	0.15	-0.06	0.44*	0.29*	-0.38*	0.00

Note: Negative values indicate rural states had lower rates than urban states. Positive values indicate they had higher rates.
* = $p < .05$.

ity rates and urbanization, we calculated Spearman rank correlation coefficients. The coefficients were obtained using the rankings for the forty-eight continental states for each disease category and each of the five time periods by gender. The results of the rank correlations show a clear trend throughout the 1939–1981 time period. For simplicity, the significant results for three of the time periods—1939–1941, 1959–1961, and 1979–1981—are provided in table 3.1.

Negative values in table 3.1 indicate that people living in rural states had lower death rates from specific causes than did those residing in urban states. In 1939–1941, white males in rural states had significantly lower age-adjusted death rates from diabetes, heart diseases, suicide, cancer, and all causes than did white males residing in urban states. White females in rural states had significantly lower rates for diabetes, heart diseases, suicide, accidents, cancer, and all causes than did their urban counterparts. The category influenza/pneumonia showed higher rates, and no significant differences were evident between white females in urban and rural states for deaths from homicide and cerebrovascular diseases.

The lower death rates experienced in rural states were not lost on researchers looking for explanations. The apparent protection of rural dwellers from high death rates helped continue the illusion that persists today—that rural living is healthy living. Another way to describe the phenomenon is to say that in 1939–1941 people in the most urbanized states paid the ultimate price for their choice of living conditions—the *urban penalty* for health.

What is most striking about table 3.1 is the change in the pattern of death over time. White females lose the protection of rural living by 1979–1981 for most causes of death—that is, the rank correlation for diabetes changes from –0.61 to –0.19, that for heart diseases from –0.66 to 0.15, that for suicide from –0.59 to 0.15, and that for cancer from –0.78 to –0.15. In fact, white women living in rural states had two significantly higher correlations with mortality than did white women living in urban states in 1979–1981: 0.31 for cerebrovascular diseases and 0.27 for influenza/pneumonia. The urban penalty, then, is no longer apparent for middle-aged white females, with women from rural states exhibiting little differences in mortality from most causes in 1979–1981, and those from rural states having significantly higher death rates from two causes—cerebrovascular diseases and influenza/pneumonia.

For white males in the 1979–1981 period, the change is even more striking. Although rural residence had a protective effect from many causes of death for white males at the state scale in 1939–1941, the effect disappears over time. In fact, for heart diseases, suicide, accidents, cancer, cerebrovascular diseases, other and all causes, white males in rural states had significantly higher age-adjusted death rates than their urban counterparts in 1979–1981 (Spearman rank correlations between death rates for these seven categories of death and percent urban: 0.38, 0.29, 0.54, 0.32, 0.48, 0.44, and 0.32, respectively). This reversal in death rates seems to suggest a new phenomenon for white males—the *rural penalty* for health.

Table 3.1 points out the fallacy of using urbanization as the key to understanding high death rates over time. Although percent urban could probably predict personal habits and behaviors that effect disease outcome in earlier time periods, today's homogeneity of culture, population migration, and other factors have eliminated urbanization as a predictor of high death rates, at least for middle-aged whites. For this population there is no longer an urban penalty; a new problem—the rural penalty—has emerged. We are currently investigating whether this pattern also holds true for other populations, such as blacks, Hispanics, and other age cohorts.

Urbanization, Poverty, and Health in Rural States

We wanted to see if we could determine whether our hypothesis was correct, that is, that poverty rather than urban status was the major force now driving high death rates. We chose the twenty-eight states that were less than 50 percent urban in 1940 and examined what happened to those states over the next forty years. If the state remained less than 50 percent urban in 1980, we categorized it as rural/rural, that is, that it was rural in 1940 and remained so in 1980. Seven states fit into the rural/rural category: Mississippi, North Dakota, South Dakota, North Carolina, West Virginia, Vermont, and Maine. Our second category consisted of states that were rural in 1940, but became moderately urban, that is, 50 percent to 64 percent urban, in 1980. Our rural/moderately urban category contained eleven states: Arkansas, South Carolina, Kentucky, Alabama, Idaho, Georgia, Tennessee, Wyoming, Montana, Nebraska, and Iowa. A third category consisted of states that were rural in 1940, but became strongly urban, that is, 65 percent or more urban, in 1980. Ten states fit into the rural/strongly urban category: New Mexico, Arizona, Virginia, Oklahoma, Nevada, Louisiana, Kansas, Texas, Oregon, and Minnesota. If urbanization was the key predictor of increased death rates for specific diseases, death rates should have increased more in the rural/urban states than the rural/rural ones or decreased less in the rural/urban than the rural/rural ones.

Using the same nine categories of disease for white males and females as were used in the Spearman correlations, we compared the average age-adjusted rates of the three groups. We created ratios that reflect how the degree of urbanization in formerly rural states is associated with mortality. Specifically, if urbanization is the key to understanding high death rates, then Group 1 states (rural in 1940 and remaining rural in 1980) should have lower average rates than Group 3 and also Group 2 states (places that were rural in 1940 but became more urban by 1980). Low ratios, those less than 1.00, reflect low rates in the more rural areas and support the notion that urbanization and high mortality rates are linked. Ratios greater than 1.00 reflect higher rates in the rural states, and refute the notion of urbanization being linked to high mortality.

Table 3.2. Comparison of Age-Adjusted Death Rates for White Males and Females (Thirty-five to Sixty-four Years Old) by Percent Urban Status and Per Capita Personal Income (1979–1981)

Group	Percent urban status			Per capita personal income		
	1 v. 2	1 v. 3	2 v. 3	1 v. 2	1 v. 3	2 v. 3
Males						
All causes	1.03	1.10	1.07	1.20	1.25	1.04
Influenza/pneumonia	0.97	0.96	0.98	1.24	1.27	1.03
Diabetes	1.14	1.06	0.93	1.06	1.14	1.08
Heart diseases	1.06	1.19	1.13	1.21	1.27	1.05
Suicide	0.94	1.02	1.08	1.05	1.05	1.00
Homicide	0.70	0.65	0.93	1.35	1.45	1.08
Accidents	0.96	1.04	1.08	1.05	1.11	1.06
Cancer	1.01	1.08	1.06	1.12	1.25	1.11
Cerebrovascular diseases	1.02	1.20	1.17	1.24	1.41	1.15
Other	1.06	1.03	0.97	1.21	1.28	1.06
Females						
All causes	1.02	1.04	1.02	1.13	1.06	0.93
Influenza/pneumonia	0.99	0.87	0.88	1.07	0.94	0.88
Diabetes	0.91	0.91	1.00	1.20	1.10	1.03
Heart diseases	1.09	1.20	1.11	1.25	1.28	1.02
Suicide	1.06	0.93	0.87	1.02	0.94	0.92
Homicide	0.80	0.62	0.85	1.32	1.11	0.84
Accidents	0.76	0.74	1.11	0.99	0.91	0.94
Cancer	1.05	1.17	1.06	1.09	1.02	0.94
Cerebrovascular diseases	1.02	1.18	1.15	1.13	1.24	1.09
Other	0.96	0.84	0.84	1.15	0.93	0.81

Key: Change in percent urban status: Group 1 = rural/rural, Group 2 = rural/moderately urban, Group 3 = rural/strongly urban. Per capita personal income: Group 1 = rural states among the lowest ten ranked for per capita personal income in 1980, Group 2 = rural states in the 20 to 50 percent range for per capita personal income in 1980, Group 3 = rural states in the greater than 50 percent range for per capita personal income in 1980.

The results, shown in table 3.2, are mixed. For example, for middle-aged white males, states that became moderately urbanized (Group 2) between 1940 and 1980 had higher rates for influenza/pneumonia (0.97), homicide (0.70), suicide (0.94), and accidents (0.96) than did states that remained rural. Males in more rural states had higher rates for diabetes (1.14), heart diseases (1.06), cancer (1.01), and cerebrovascular diseases (1.02).

For middle-aged white females, Group 2 states that became more urban had higher rates for influenza/pneumonia (0.99), diabetes (0.91), homicide (0.80), and accidents (0.76). Females in more rural states had higher rates of heart diseases (1.09), suicide (1.06), cancer (1.05), and cerebrovascular diseases (1.02).

Using the sixty possible comparisons (three group comparisons and ten disease categories for each gender), the change in percent urban status yielded ratios of average mortality ranks that were higher for places that became more urban in twenty-five instances, were lower in thirty-four, and exhibited no change in one. These results simply confirm what was determined by the Spearman correlations. Urbanization is no longer a good predictor of high death rates.

As the second step of testing our hypothesis, we examined the changing relationship between age-adjusted death rates and poverty. We used the same twenty-eight states that were rural in 1940, but this time we categorized them by their per capita personal income levels in 1980. That is, we wished to know whether per capita personal income was a good predictor of high death rates in the 1979–1981 period.

Three groups were formed representing different income levels. Group 1 consisted of nine rural states that fell into the lowest ten ranked continental states for per capita personal income in 1980: Mississippi, Arkansas, South Carolina, Alabama, Kentucky, Tennessee, West Virginia, Maine, and North Carolina. Group 2 contained twelve rural states, those that fell within the twenty to fifty percent range of continental states ranked for per capita personal income in 1980: Vermont, New Mexico, South Dakota, Idaho, Georgia, Montana, Louisiana, North Dakota, Arizona, Nebraska, Oklahoma, and Virginia. The third group had seven rural states and represented those that were among the top fifty percent of states for per capita personal income in 1980: Iowa, Oregon, Texas, Minnesota, Kansas, Nevada, and Wyoming.

We again calculated ratios. The results of this effort are found in the right columns of table 3.2. Ratios exceeding 1.0 mean that the poorer states had higher death rates than the more affluent states. Ratios less than 1.0 mean that the more affluent states had higher death rates.

The ratios of per capita personal income in table 3.2 show startling results. Males living in the poorest states have markedly higher ratios for all ten categories of death. Furthermore, every ratio comparing the poorest to wealthiest rural states (1 versus 3 in the right columns) is higher than the corresponding ratio comparing mortality in the most rural to now heavily urban states (1 versus 3 in the left columns). Of all possible ratios comparing male rates by per capita personal income in rural states, all thirty are over 1.00. These results plainly show the relationship of poverty and higher death rates for middle-aged white males in more rural states in the 1979–1981 period.

For white females, those living in the poorest rural states (based on per capita personal income for 1980) have higher death rates for all causes except accidents than those living in rural states with somewhat higher per capita personal incomes. Women living in the most wealthy states (those that were rural in 1940, but which now are in the greater than 50 percent range for per capita personal income) show higher ratios for diabetes, heart diseases, and cerebrovascular diseases as causes of death. Over all thirty possible comparisons (three group comparisons and ten disease categories), white women in the poorer rural states had higher death rates in eighteen instances, lower rates in twelve. Per capita personal income does predict mortality rates, but not quite as well for middle-aged white females as for males. It is most useful for predicting high rates for women in all death categories except accidents in the poorest of the rural states.

The results we obtained are so striking that we feel it prudent to offer explanations for the patterns observed. One credible set of explanations for these findings can be drawn from studies of behavioral risks. Surveys show that, while sedentary lifestyles are less of a problem for rural residents than urban ones, rural male smoking rates are significantly higher than those for urban males, especially among the middle-aged and elderly. This may partially explain the higher rates of cancer and heart disease among rural males (Greenberg, 1987b).

Rural states also have a greater prevalence of obesity and higher rates of hypertension than do urban states. New Jersey males and females, for instance, had hypertension rates of 2.8 and 4.5 percent, respectively, in 1981. North Carolina reported hypertension rates of 4.2 and 7.1 percent for the same time period. Behavioral risk factor surveys show, in general, that urban residents now exhibit healthier behaviors than rural residents (Greenberg, 1987b). This leaves rural states with two strikes against them—both poverty and the increased personal risks taken by their inhabitants.

Personal risk-taking behaviors are highly correlated with educational level. The relationship between smoking and educational achievement is particularly noteworthy. Centers for Disease Control and state behavioral risk surveys show that smoking among the least educated young people (those with less than a ninth-grade education) was three times that of those with a college education (55 percent to 19 percent) and almost twice that of those with some high school (55 percent to 37 percent) in 1981. In contrast, among those with the most years of formal education, only 5 percent smoked (Greenberg, 1987b). The implications of these findings are significant for rural inhabitants. Although the educational achievement of those in rural areas has increased in recent years, as late as 1987 it still fell behind that of the average urbanite (O'Hare, 1988). In that year, 20 percent of young rural adults did not finish high school. The corresponding figure was less than 15 percent for urban residents. Given these findings, it is likely that health problems from smoking will continue to be higher among rural inhabitants for many years.

Rural residents who do finish high school and go on to college are likely to move to urban areas permanently. This leaves the overall level of education in rural areas low, resulting in higher levels of unemployment. These higher unemployment levels then translate into poverty status for many rural Americans. For workers who dropped out of high school, the 1986 poverty rate was 24 percent for rural areas compared to 20 percent in urban areas (O'Hare, 1988).

The pattern becomes more complex because rural states often have more restrictive welfare eligibility rules and fewer benefits. Families that stay together are ineligible for the major welfare program, Aid to Families with Dependent Children in nearly half the states. Those living on family farms are ineligible for benefits because they fail to meet the "assets test." Rural inhabitants, then, are in general more likely to have low educational achievement, be unemployed, and live in poverty status than are urbanites. Rural residents are also less likely to qualify for public assistance because of eligibility requirements and more likely to take more personal risks than are their urban counterparts (O'Hare, 1988). This cycle has dire implications for the health of rural Americans—especially poor rural Americans—and the effects are only starting to be measured.

The National Health Interview Survey (U.S. National Center for Health Statistics, 1984) reports the health status of persons by age, sex, race, income, geographic region, and location of residence. In 1980, residents of rural areas (that is, people outside an MSA) were more likely to report their health as fair or poor than were urban residents (14.2 percent and 11.1 percent, respectively). The same data, restructured for family income, show that persons in the lowest income group felt their health was fair to poor 22.5 percent of the time. Only 6.5 percent in the highest income group reported poor health. Combining rural status with poverty, then, yields the worst of both worlds. It leaves many of the rural poor with little hope for good health.

The inequality in health status between low- and high-income groups has been explained by lack of access to health care. How much can really be attributed to poor access? Starr (1981) claims very little, as the 1970s saw a significant movement toward equalization in the use of medical services in the United States. The poor actually now have more physician visits per year than the affluent (5.5 to 4.6 in 1980) and have longer lengths of stay in hospitals (8.4 days to 6.0 days in 1980) (U.S. National Center for Health Statistics, 1984; see chapter 1 for more on physician visits).

Focusing efforts on equalizing access to medical care without addressing the underlying social problems of poverty will not alleviate major gaps in health status between the rich and the poor. The true problem is simply that the poor are less healthy and more prone to chronic illnesses (Starr, 1981). Often this is because of poorer diets, poorer living conditions and increased personal risk-taking behaviors over a lifetime. Simply opening the doors to medical care once health problems are apparent will not reduce the health status gap. By then it is frequently too late.

Poverty as the New Driving Factor for Death Rates in Rural Areas

Although the health status of low-income groups in the United States has improved over the past three decades, people in poverty still experience more than their share of illness and death. Whether poverty accounts for ill health or ill health causes poverty has been an ongoing debate over the years. What is clear, however, is that low income remains statistically linked to both poor health status and excess mortality (Dutton, 1986). The working poor, blacks, Hispanics, migrant farm workers, the homeless, and rural residents in general all experience significant excesses in mortality from cancer, heart diseases and stroke, cirrhosis, diabetes, homicides/accidents, and infant mortality (U.S. Department of Health and Human Services, 1985a,b). These groups are not highly visible or vocal, and their situation is not improving with time.

Media coverage of the unrest in the 1960s linked poverty to the urban ghetto. The fact of the matter, however, is that today it is rural America that is experiencing growing levels of economic distress. In 1986, fifty-four million Americans lived in rural areas and 18 percent of them lived in poverty, a rate approximately 50 percent higher than that for urban areas. In addition, one out of every four children in rural areas lived in poverty in that year and unemployment was 26 percent higher than in urban areas (O'Hare, 1988; see chapter 1 for more details on poverty and unemployment). Clearly, the current economic situation for rural Americans is bleak.

With the failure of many farms over the last decade, population movement out of small towns has increased as the young and able-bodied move to suburban and urban areas looking for work. Those too poor and undereducated to move are left behind, victims of the deteriorating rural economy. Many of those left behind are now homeless. Indeed, the rural poor account for up to 90 percent of the homeless in states such as South Dakota (*New York Times*, 1989).

Many of the rural poor do not receive public assistance, do not live in public housing, do not receive food stamps, are not covered by Medicaid, and do not have access to medical care (D. Rowland and Lyons, 1989). P. A. Butler (1988) suggests that rural feelings against receiving aid, embarrassment, and lack of information and/or local resources accounts for some of this. Yet this explanation seems too stereotypical and too easy to use as justification for government inaction. The lack of both public and private services has serious implications for the health and resultant death rates of rural Americans. The isolated rural poor need to be educated about their diets, alcoholism, cigarette smoking, and other behavioral risks. They need to learn about work-related and environmental contamination risks at least as much as their inner-city counterparts. To achieve these ends both government and private help is needed to provide the resources and opportunities required for the rural poor to take advantage of these educational experiences.

Conclusion

The convergence phenomenon resulting from our increasing homogeneity of lifestyles from the 1930s through the 1960s had a tendency to drive death rates toward a national norm. Now the rapidly increasing poverty in rural areas, first evident during the 1970s and 1980s, is driving some mortality rates farther from their urban counterparts. The rural penalty for health has emerged as a new phenomenon, at least for middle-aged whites. Only further investigation will show whether this is also true for other age and racial/ethnic cohorts.

Urbanization and poverty offer competing explanations for mortality trends in the United States. We have examined U.S. death rates over the past forty years and suggest that using one or the other as the sole explanation of these trends will lead researchers to erroneous conclusions. The social realities of each time period under study need to be considered if we are to understand patterns of death. Poverty and rural America are today linked closely, perhaps inextricably.

Chapter 4

Implications of Changing Demographic Structures for Rural Health Services

MELINDA S. MEADE

The term "rural" is a broad one. It encompasses farm and non-farm, lands contiguous to great metropolises and lands remote from any town, places of economic growth and those of decline, places of retirement and those of abandonment. Such differences are associated with differences in demographic structure, that is, the proportions of different ages, races, and sexes. Since age, race, and sex are characterized by different levels of risk of various morbidity or mortality conditions, great variation in need for services in "rural" America exists. In this chapter, I try to show some variations of service need associated with age, sex, and race, and offer a typology of rural regions based on demographic differentiation. I conclude with a discussion of some implications of local population projections and changing structural context.

Morbidity and Mortality Have Demographic Parameters

"Stage of life" is a convenient rubric to summarize the experiences, needs, and characteristics of the human condition. Although there is a broadly shared human experience, variations by ethnicity and race have real implications for morbidity and mortality. Unless otherwise noted, all the data used in this section come from the U.S. National Center for Health Statistics (NCHS), *Monthly Vital Statistics Report 1987* (1989) on mortality statistics.

Infancy

Until almost the age of sixty years, the greatest risk of dying occurs during the first year after birth. Deaths under one year are in turn concentrated in the neonatal period under one month. "Certain conditions originating in the perinatal period" lead all causes. The chief components are respiratory conditions and distress, and disorders related to short gestation and low birth weight. Congenital abnormalities, especially of the heart and respiratory system, are the second cause. Sudden infant death syndrome, accidents, and pneumonia complete the five leading causes. There is considerable variation between the races, although whites and blacks both share those rankings. Sudden infant death syndrome is almost twice as common among blacks (120.5 : 225.5), accidents are twice as common (21.7 : 42.4), and pneumonia is more than twice as common (13.6 : 35.2). Black infant deaths from homicide (17.0) are more common than white infant deaths from pneumonia. The most striking racial differences, however, lie in conditions originating in the perinatal period, especially those relating to short gestation and low birth weight (59.4 : 233.2)

These differences have attracted considerable research, cause by cause and influence by influence. Birth weight has emerged as a crucial variable. Eberstein and Parker (1984) used linked birth and death records from a 1975 cohort and found that the impact of birth weight is more important than that of maternal age on infant mortality. Carlson (1984) found a serious, but rather enigmatic, racial gap existing in the odds of low birth weight. Working in South Carolina, he could not explain the high incidence of low birth weight among blacks as a result of black-white differences in age or education of mothers, prenatal care, parity, or length of birth interval. Although these were all predictors of birth weight, the tendency to have low birth weights persisted even after they were controlled. Age, parity, and birth order affected the odds of low birth weight for blacks and whites in the same way, but education and prenatal care did not cause nearly so steep a decline in the odds among blacks as whites. This is troubling to those who, like Williams and Chen (1982), see improvement in birth weights as holding the greatest promise for future reduction in infant deaths.

Death rates from human immunodeficiency virus (HIV) among infants are rising rapidly and becoming more differentiated by race. Even in 1987 rates were 9.4 per 100,000 for blacks, 7.5 for Hispanics, and 1.1 for whites.

Childhood

Since fatal infectious disease in children has been largely eliminated through vaccination and antibiotics, the major cause of death is accidents and even these barely rise to 20 per 100,000 among small children. Cancer, especially leukemia, does occur and congenital anomalies still take their toll, especially in heart disease. Pneumonia and meningitis do kill, rarely, but murder is more common and, among whites, suicide. There is little racial difference in cause of death except that, among blacks and Hispanics, HIV has become one of the top ten causes of death.

Young Adulthood

Violence—accidents, homicide, and suicide—accounts for 76 percent of deaths among those aged fifteen to twenty-four. Cancer, followed by heart disease and congenital abnormalities, continues to be important, but HIV has moved into next place (at 1.3 percent). The death rate from all causes barely reaches 99 per 100,000. This overall rate is deceptive, however, because of the great gender difference created by violent death (see table 4.1).

Maturity

During the mature years from twenty-five to sixty-four years, death rates increase from 100 to almost 900 per 100,000, degenerative diseases rise to dominance, and gender, racial, and ethnic differentials increase. Overall, black males continue to have by far the highest death rates, with a differential over white males that increases from 100 to 1000 with age. White females have the lowest death rates over this period, about half those of black females and ranging from only 17 percent to 35 percent of black male rates.

Between early and late maturity, accidents fall from first to fourth cause of death, suicide from fourth to eighth, and homicide from fifth to tenth. Cancer becomes the major cause of death, followed by heart disease and cerebrovascular disease. Lung disease, liver disease, and diabetes mellitus similarly move up. Male

Table 4.1. Deaths per 100,000 by Age, Race, and Sex (1987)

Age	White males	White females	Black males	Black females
<1	942.1	742.8	2,211.4	1,781.5
1–4	52	40.54	90.5	73.5
5–9	27.4	17.9	39.1	27.1
10–14	32.8	17.9	46.1	22.7
15–19	116.3	48.7	144.2	49.0
20–24	156.9	49.5	266.9	86.2
25–29	156.4	56.4	327.4	118.0
30–34	179.5	68.8	458.4	184.3
35–39	218.4	96.8	631.5	250.8
40–44	286.8	145.5	798.0	357.0
45–49	445.4	248.1	1,041.9	513.6
50–54	738.9	412.4	1,515.3	796.1
55–59	1,198.5	650.0	1,995.3	1,131.8
60–64	1,920.2	1,044.2	2,986.8	1,786.4
65–69	2,836.6	1,589.1	4,061.7	2,401.8
70–74	4,504.1	2,497.6	5,703.6	3,485.3
75–79	6,865.4	3,963.8	7,869.4	4,939.3
80–84	10,671.7	6,745.8	12,045.5	8,335.7
≥85	18,434.9	14,486.9	15,226.1	12,312.2

Source: U.S. National Center for Health Statistics (1989).

death rates are more than twice female rates for ischemic heart disease, emphysema, and lung cancer; but equal with lung cancer in women is death from breast cancer.

Until this stage of life, cause of death was very similar across racial and ethnic groups except that whites are more prone to suicide and blacks and Hispanics to homicide. Other differences now appear. Chronic pulmonary obstructive disease (mainly emphysema) is the fourth cause of deaths for whites in late maturity, but only the eighth cause for blacks (although at only slightly lower rates), and only tenth for Hispanics. From thirty-five to forty-four, white male death rates from HIV are 21.7, those for black males 72.9. The third-ranking cause of death among Hispanics is liver disease, and the sixth is diabetes; among whites, these rank sixth and eighth, respectively. Despite shifts in ranking importance, however, the top ten causes of death are the same for all three groups except for the continuing importance of suicide for whites and murder for blacks and Hispanics.

Seniority

The mortality curve begins to climb steeply as seniority (ages sixty-five to seventy-four) is entered. Heart disease and cancer are, of course, the major causes of death. They account for 75 percent of deaths in this stage, so that even a small decline in the incidence of heart disease can add years to life expectancy, as happened recently. Cerebrovascular disease, mostly stroke, is the third cause for all groups. Chronic obstructive pulmonary diseases are next in importance for whites but lower than diabetes for others. Kidney disease becomes one of the ten major causes of death. Death rates from chronic liver disease and cirrhosis peak in this stage. The rate of suicide, which has been on a plateau for decades, begins to rise, whereas homicide reaches its lowest level. Fatal infections increase markedly, mostly from pneumonia but also septicemia; although at much lower rates than the top ten causes, deaths from tuberculosis also increase and those from viral hepatitis peak. Overall, the causes of mortality become remarkably similar, although blacks continue to have death rates half again as high as whites, and male deaths to exceed female.

The risk of functional disability increases rapidly after age sixty-five. Although three-quarters of seniors have no difficulty with such personal care activities as walking, bathing, getting outside, getting out of a chair, or dressing, 9.1 percent of those aged seventy to seventy-four have trouble with at least one personal care activity and 4.2 percent with more than four of them (U.S. National Center for Health Statistics, 1989). Even by age eighty-five, however, only half of people have difficulty with one activity (mostly walking), and fewer than one in five elderly have difficulty with more than four.

Old Age

The causes of death in old age merely reflect escalating rates of the causes in seniority, except that pneumonia increases in importance. Morbidity, however, increases greatly. More than half the population suffers from arthritis; roughly a third suffers from cataracts or serious impairment of vision (more among females) and from hearing impairment (more among males) (U.S. National Center for Health Statistics, 1989). Although the average age of death is rising, the average period spent disabled may be increasing (Soldo and Agree, 1988).

Those over eighty-five, although a small portion of the population, are the most rapidly growing segment. They are characterized by their uniquely low sex ratio (there being few males per female), high rates of institutionalization, low family income, and low proportion of minorities (Manton and Soldo, 1985; Rosenwaike, 1985). They are also characterized by markedly higher rates of mental disease, which Kramer (1980) has characterized as a "rising pandemic of mental disorders." Manton and Stallard (1982) have suggested that as deaths owing to disease processes decrease and more people approach the genetically given biological limits of life, chronic disease could become "rectangularized," or persist at high levels after onset for the duration of longer lives.

Changing Experience

In chapter 3 of this book the convergence of death rates and the role of poverty are discussed. It must simply be noted here that twenty years from now some of these stage-of-life associations may no longer hold. Mortality and morbidity are subject to a strong cohort effect: the different life experience of people born years apart changes their patterns of ill health. "Multiple-cause-of-death" reporting systems and recent demographic techniques of "decomposing" changes in life expectancy and allocating risk of death from elimination of specific diseases at various ages has allowed mortality differentials to be examined by sex, ethnicity, region, and other subpopulations (Manton and Stallard, 1982; Arriaga, 1984; Pollard, 1988). Targeting specific conditions or behaviors in specific populations for intervention or special service will thus be possible. Such programs could alter the ethnicity and age patterns described earlier.

As the custom of smoking cigarettes declines, for example, it becomes unlikely that lung cancer will again reach its previous level of prevalence overall; however, it is presently increasing among females even as it declines among males because of changes in smoking behavior. Changing attitudes toward cholesterol, exercise, and how many children are desirable will affect future disease and death statistics. HIV is a new player on the field of life. Gene therapy and abortion of fetuses with serious congenital abnormalities may greatly lower neonatal death rates. The difference in life expectancy between the sexes, which had been widening since 1900, decreased by a year in the past decade, to 6.9 years (78.4 for females compared to 71.5 for males). In April of 1990 the Census Bureau announced that for the first time in many decades the sex ratio for each decade had increased (i.e., there were more males per 100 females), partly owing to in-migration but mostly to declining male mortality from heart disease and lung cancer. The difference in life expectancy between blacks and whites narrowed from 7.6 years in 1970 to 5.6 years in 1983–1984; then black life expectancy actually declined during 1984–1986 while white life expectancy increased slightly so that the divergence again exceeds 6.2 years (75.6 and 69.4 in 1987). Over the next decade it is possible that public health education could change behavior and lower risk for diabetes, lung cancer, cardiovascular disease, motor vehicle accidents, alcoholism and drug abuse, low birth weight, and death from handguns. Any such changes would greatly affect the life-stage patterns of morbidity and mortality, especially for minority populations.

For one thing, the present relationship of poverty and low socioeconomic status and limited access to health care may change as the structure for funding health care changes. Currently, need and demand for health services may differ and bias the statistical pattern. From 1971 to 1981, for example, Mexican-Americans are reported to have suffered excess deaths, compared to the general population, not only from external causes such as motor vehicle accidents and homicide, but also because their rates of diabetes were three times those for whites, and because they suffered the highest relative risk of tuberculosis in the country (U.S. Department of Health and Human Services, 1985a,b). Yet Mexican-Americans were also described as having a health status closer to whites than blacks, with low reported functional disability rates, low infant mortality, and low cardiovascular disease. Richichi addressed the question of whether the relatively lower use of health services by Hispanics was due to limitation of access or to better health on the part of selected migrants. After analyzing generational data from the NHANES national survey, she concluded that the low use of medical services was a consequence of poor socioeconomic status and inability to afford care (Richichi, 1988). A change in the national system of paying for preventive health services, especially, might have a major impact on the disease associations of various life stages.

Spatial Patterns

There is great spatial variation in mortality across the United States. Some of this variation is due to disease ecology. There are, for example, important differences in dietary patterns or spatially distinct religious groups, in frequency of atmospheric inversion and pollution, in unemployment, or in presence of radiation sources. One major cause for the variation, however, is demographic structure.

The dimensions of differences in mortality are striking. Consider the following contrasts in the ratio of death rates for five causes (table 4.2). Michigan is a heavily industrialized state of out-migration and Texas one of the most rapidly growing states; Massachusetts is the most metropolitan state, and South Carolina one of the most rural; the highest and lowest state for the nation or for the contiguous forty-eight states are often dramatically different.

The threefold difference in deaths from cancer between Florida and Alaska is simply explained by the difference in age structure between a state of high in-migration of seniors and one that receives young adults. The low rates of Utah are likely ecological, owing to the different cultural behavior of Mormons. The differences in accidental death between the most unforgiving environment and the most benign (with the least road distance) are understandable, but those between the rural expanses of New

Table 4.2. Ratios of Death Rates for Five Causes across States (1985)

Cause	MI/TX	MA/SC	Highest/lowest
Cancer	1.3	1.3	3.3 (FL/AK); 2.7 (FL/UT)
Accidents	1.2	1.6	3.2 (AK/HI); 2.1 (NM/RI)
Chronic liver and cirrhosis	1.7	1.3	3.1 (NY/ID)
Homicide	1.1	0.4	7.9 (TX/NH)
Suicide	0.9	0.8	3.3 (WY/NY)

Note: Where two values are given for highest/lowest, the first value is for the nation as a whole and the second is for the contiguous forty-eight states.
Source: Calculated from U.S. National Center for Health Statistics reported data.

Mexico and the urban ones of Rhode Island raise other questions. The fact that Texans are eight times more likely to be murdered than people in New Hampshire cannot be explained by age structure; Texas ranks forty-seventh in percent of state population over the age of sixty-five, but New Hampshire ranks only thirty-third. Differences in ethnicity are involved, but the magnitude of the difference suggests fundamental differences in social pathology. Similarly, the threefold difference in suicide between Wyoming and New York cannot be explained by age structure, as Wyoming has one of the lowest proportions of seniors and elderly. Ethnicity may be involved, as states with high proportions of nonwhites tend to have lower suicide rates, but Wyoming's rate is also twice those of Nebraska and Iowa. The metropolitan and industrial states have higher rates of cancer, alcohol damage, and (mostly motor vehicle) accidents, but lower rates of suicide. The first two are in the right direction for positive correlation with ages, but accident and suicide rates run counter to that pattern and have a more detailed ecology.

The differences in age, sex, and ethnicity between states and the different risks of exposure that in-migration brings to the destination's statistics on disease have far-reaching implications for varying needs for health services. As the population proceeds through its stages of life, needs such as those for obstetrical services, dialysis, or long-term care for mental impairment, or preventive health education change. In this way not only are rural areas differentiated from urban, but it is also important to differentiate rural areas by types of migration and by age structure.

Variations among States and Counties

The projected growth in the elderly population is not going to be expressed with spatial uniformity. First, there will be different proportions of elderly depending on local marriage and fertility behavior. Second, the importance of "aging" in place will vary depending on the out-migration of young adults. Third, the proportion of elderly in some places will be driven by selective in-migration of retirees or, increasingly over time, of the aged.

The rural population as a whole, and its farm and nonfarm components, is demographically distinctive to begin with, according to information from Current Population Reports (U.S. Department of Commerce, Bureau of the Census, and U.S. Department of Agriculture, Economic Research Service, 1988). Whereas the median age of the urban population in 1987 was 31.8 years, that of the rural nonfarm population was 32.0 and that of the rural farm population, 37.6. Farm families are more likely than nonfarm families to have both husband and wife present (94 percent versus 80 percent) and to have higher levels of childbearing (2,031 children born per 1,000 ever-married women eighteen to forty-four years of age, compared with 1,781 children per 1,000 nonfarm women), but less likely to have children living at home (41 percent versus 50 percent). Since 1920 the ratio of males to females has been higher in the farm population (in 1987, 109 for the farm population and 93 for the nonfarm population). Despite the higher sex ratio, a slightly higher percentage of the farm population is in the late mature and senior stages, and more of the nonfarm population in the young adult, early mature, and childhood stages.

The diversity created by aging and migration is great. For example, the five states with the largest numbers of persons aged sixty-five and over are California, New York, Florida, Pennsylvania, and Texas; those with the largest percentage of their population aged sixty-five and over, in order, are Florida, Pennsylvania, Rhode Island, Iowa, and Arkansas; those with the greatest percentage increase in that group over the period 1980–1986 are Alaska, Nevada, Hawaii, Arizona, and New Mexico. The largest states will have the greatest demands for beds and services for the diseases of maturity and old age, but some of the central states with past out-migration will bear a heavier burden of aging, and some of the smaller states, the greatest relative change in demand for resources.

The 1980 Census showed a great increase in the percentage of single-person households—young unmarried people, divorced, widowed—and dramatized the big surprise: for the first time, the pattern of rural-to-urban migration was reversed and metropolitan areas were losing population while rural areas grew. In the late 1980s, there seemed to be a decline in this counter-urbanization marked by a dramatic decrease in the ability of nonmetropolitan counties to retain population (Elo and Beale, 1988). The 1990 Census found that one-quarter of the American population now lives alone. Many of the rural counties that had grown, especially the coal mining and petroleum prospecting ones, lost population over the last decade (U.S. Department of Commerce, Bureau of the Census, 1991).

Broad generalizations about nonmetropolitan conditions and trends can conceal important diversity (Brown and Beale, 1981). The counter-urbanization movement and the movement to the Sunbelt were analyzed into numerous typologies and associations (Little, 1980; Brown and Beale, 1981; Airola and Parker, 1983; Lichter et al., 1985; Morrill, 1988). The movement to nonmetropolitan areas was not merely increasing urban sprawl, although that did occur. It was movement to rural areas noncontiguous with metropolitan areas. Growth occurred mainly in places with populations of under 2,500 people, which accounted for 30 percent of absolute national growth (although 66 percent of absolute national growth still occurred in metropolitan areas). The trend of past decades, concentration at national scale and deconcentration locally, ended and the country deconcentrated nationally. There were three major types of nonmetropolitan destinations. Places related to energy development (such as new or newly revived coal mining, petroleum exploration, or oil shale exploitation) and to some extent mineral extraction were booming then—although many have now collapsed. Recreational destinations on coasts, lakes, and mountains were attracting the working people needed to make them go. Most importantly, people were retiring to new areas. Industries were also decentralizing and moving plants, but often to new metropolitan areas, such as those in North Carolina, Tennessee, Wisconsin, and Texas. The migrations for retirement and recreational development were clearly affected by climate, distinctive lifestyle (New Hampshire, New Mexico), and presence of water bodies. Since most retired people stay where they are or migrate only locally, however, not only the south and southwest grew from retirement migration. There were large influxes of seniors to the upper peninsula of Michigan, Missouri, Oregon, and Arkansas, as well as substantial increases in the senior and elderly population of the industrialized northeast.

There were modest changes during this period in racial distribution across residential categories, as blacks were underrepresented in deconcentration (Lichter et al., 1986). Like whites in earlier years, blacks tended to move to suburbs rather than noncontiguous rural areas. Cromartie (1990) has shown, however, that the return migration of blacks to the south is not limited to retirees and that it has a substantial rural destination component. The

Chicano population remained highly metropolitan (Tienda, 1981). Despite the nonmetropolitan retirement destinations of the 1970s, the elderly during the period 1960–1980 became more highly concentrated spatially and more urban. As higher incomes and longer periods of retirement became common, the elderly increasingly favored large towns over sparsely settled counties (McCarthy, 1983).

There is evidence of both continuance and change in these patterns. From 1965–1970 to 1980–1985 gross and net migration flows have persisted: the northeast "core," for example, has lost to all other regions, and the northwest "periphery" has gained from all other regions, while Florida and California have continued their extraordinary growth (Morrill, 1988). Nonmetropolitan areas mainly characterized by primary sector activities (agriculture and mining) have experienced widespread decline in the last few years, although retirement areas have not (Elo and Beale, 1988). For decades, "aging-in-place" has accounted for much of the growth in proportion of the elderly of a typical county, although this was strongly influenced by out-migration of the young in the 1950s and 1960s. This process of aging has slowed markedly in recent years, and now fertility rates contribute little to spatial variation in aging (Clifford et al., 1983). Migration has come to be a much more important factor in the recent aging of counties.

A Demographic Typology of Counties

These population trends have a differential impact on the health care needs of counties. The shifts in age structure and, to some extent, cohort effects can be summarized in a typology as follows and illustrated in the population pyramids of fig. 4.1. *Aging* counties (Smith County, Kansas) are developing in place, as it were. With low fertility rates in recent years, the population is shifting gradually through higher and higher age categories. *Previous out-migration* of the young in earlier decades has left the population of some counties top-heavy in old age dependency but with a more normal age distribution as the elderly pass on (Evangeline County, Louisiana). Today out-migration of the young is creating these conditions in new areas, but they are mainly metropolitan. In-migration of young adults characterizes *booming* counties (Sweetwater County, Wyoming). The importance of the health conditions of the elderly in such places is relatively reduced, but the demand for services by childbirth and infants can be suddenly overwhelming. Finally, counties targeted as *retirement* destinations can change very rapidly, especially in absolute need (Marion County, Florida). These examples are developed more fully in the following section.

Aging counties like Smith become almost rectangular in their demographic structure. Whether they are predominantly white or black, the most important aspect of their changing health service needs is their predictability. The increase in diabetes, strokes, emphysema, and other conditions of the transition from senior to elderly can be clearly projected; the demand for obstetrics and other fertility services is constant. Programs targeting prevention of cardiovascular disease may change future sex ratios, but the preponderance of females (and so of breast cancer and other female afflictions) is clearly set. Facilities built to serve particular needs will have almost identical demand ten years later.

Previous migration counties like Evangeline are harder to interpret. A generation of young blacks, with males predominating, migrated to northern cities. The population was truncated, and people in late maturity who would soon be demanding senior health care are simply not there. It is possible that in retirement, or when they become elderly, they will return to be with family but that is too uncertain a factor to plan for. The population that remained continued its ordinary fertility behavior, with the result that the young adult population today is substantial (although fertility has fallen, as it has nationally, in recent years to decrease the proportion of children). Over the next few years the need for obstetric, pediatric, and related services will increase. Infant mortality will be a prime concern in the poor, rural county, and prevention programs will need to target birth weight issues. HIV will become increasingly important, as will homicide and accidents. There will be little relative demand for treating the conditions associated with seniors or elderly groups, although age-specific rates of afflictions are likely to be higher than in many other counties (because of the percentage of black and poor).

Booming counties such as Sweetwater are the most difficult to plan for because their permanence is uncertain. In-migration of young-mature people is attracted by the extractive industry, which can contract rapidly as it faces economic fluctuations. Although young couples and their children form a major part of the demographic impact, there are more young men coming to work than female. The health services for the elderly are likely to be neglected because they are so relatively unimportant. Suicide, homicide, and accidents will

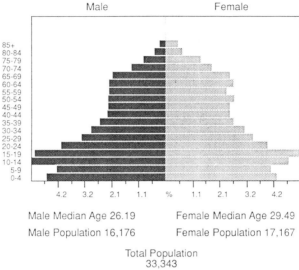

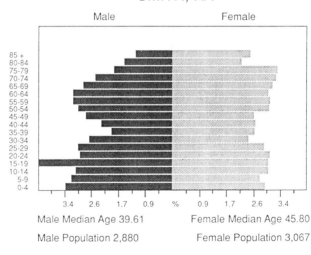

Fig. 4.1. Population pyramids for four representative counties.

SWEETWATER, WY

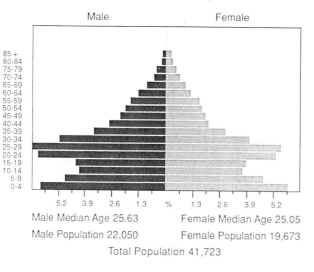

Male Median Age 25.63   Female Median Age 25.05

Male Population 22,050   Female Population 19,673

Total Population 41,723

MARION, FL

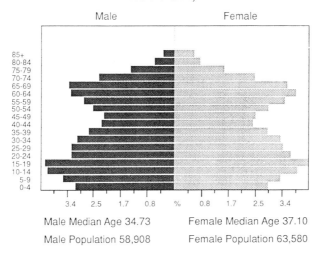

Male Median Age 34.73   Female Median Age 37.10

Male Population 58,908   Female Population 63,580

Total Population 122,488

Fig. 4.1. *(continued)*

stretch the emergency services; HIV infection will become a serious problem; gynecology and pediatrics will be services in high demand. Expensive facilities built to serve this young population, however, may find that demand for their services has evaporated in the face of high out-migration the next year.

Retirement counties are deceptive in their health care demands. On one hand, the health care needs of the senior and elderly, predominantly white population are clear and predictable. Yet variation is introduced by disease ecology, since these people were exposed to disease risk factors in another part of the country and do not necessarily continue the past health concerns of the county. Former rural cotton mill counties or mining counties, for example, may be used to lung conditions that are not typical of the in-migrant retirees. The different ethnic composition and occupational experience of the population may be reflected in the types of cancer or types of functional disabilities. The appearance of retirement in-migration may sometimes be sudden and unpredicted, but, once established, new seniors usually replace deceased or out-migrant elderly in a way conducive to planning continuing health services. One of the most rapidly increasing of these demands is for home health care and aid for functional disabilities short of full institutionalization. This, in turn, is part of the demand for services that is reflected in the lower part of the pyramid. From restaurants and shopping to grounds maintenance and health care, retirement areas require a substantial young-mature population to service them, and these people in turn have children, although proportionately fewer young ones. Demands for high schools often increase, and so do accidents and violent deaths. The least represented ages of the population are those in their late forties and fifties, who have the lowest demand for specific types of health care. As the black population has followed whites to the suburbs, one can suspect in the future there will be an increased presence of blacks in retirement areas and thus an increased importance of their health conditions (such as diabetes and hypertension).

Even while they gain overall from in-migration of other age groups, many rural counties continue to lose young adults to economic opportunities elsewhere. Although this may remove some violence and accidents, it also removes the population least subject to chronic and degenerative diseases and those able to provide some of the health care services being increasingly demanded.

Conclusion

The health care needs of rural counties reflect great demographic complexity. There are regional and local variations in this country in the proportion of population that is white, black, Hispanic, or of other ethnicity. There are great variations in age structure caused by out-, in-, and lack of migration. As a result of age and migration, there are variations in the proportion of females in each age category and overall. Each of these types of demographic variation is associated with different causes of mortality, morbidity, and dysfunction. Each has implications for planning health care services that are not served by aggregate descriptions and generalities. It is, however, possible to categorize, regionalize, and predict them and related changes in the near future.

This diversity also has importance for analysis of disease patterns. Use of county rates for analysis of disease causation or change can be strongly biased by migration. Not only does migration introduce risk and consequent conditions actually experienced elsewhere, as is widely recognized, but it also strongly affects demographic structure and can lead to the relative dominance of working or retired groups, or genders, or ethnic groups, which can hide or overwhelm local disease importance and associations. Researchers frequently acknowledge and bemoan the fact that population mobility may be affecting their causal analysis, and may decline to do such an analysis altogether. It is possible, however, to regionalize the mobility effects and maintain a comparative framework.

Counties where the population is aging in place are the kindest to those who would plan health services. Growth can benefit the provision of health care when it has been limited by small numbers and the lack of economies of scale. Decline can benefit the provision of health care when it removes demographic groups with special or intense needs. A stable rural health care system, furthermore, has functional importance in maintaining viable social systems and nurturing community (Rosenblatt, 1981). But it is most difficult to plan for or maintain where population is unstable.

PART TWO

HIGH-RISK POPULATIONS

Chapter 5

Issues in the Provision of In-Home Health Services to the Rural Elderly

An Ontario Perspective

ALUN E. JOSEPH

Statistics Canada (1984) projects an elderly (over 65) population of over 3 million (or 13.5 percent of all Canadians) by 2001 and one of over 5 million (or 24 percent of all Canadians) by 2031. The dependency ratio (the average number of people that each member of the labor force supports) in Canada will not change dramatically over the years to 2031, but the "center of gravity" of the dependent population will shift from the young to the old (Health and Welfare Canada, 1989; McDaniel, 1986). It is this supplanting of pediatrics by geriatrics that will underlie a fundamental transformation of Canada's society and institutions in the coming decades. This chapter considers the implications, over both the short and the long terms, of population aging for the provision of in-home services to the rural elderly in the Province of Ontario.

"Home care" (broadly defined to include a range of health services delivered to, and consumed in, the home) has emerged as an increasingly viable and attractive alternative to the institutionalization of elderly Canadians in need of assisted living (Chappell, 1987; National Advisory Council on Aging, 1986; Neysmith, 1988; Wallace et al., 1984). In Ontario, as in other Canadian jurisdictions, the emergence of in-home health services as a preferred strategy for meeting the needs of ailing or frail elderly persons has been encouraged on the one hand by the well-established desire of the elderly to be maintained in their own homes as long as possible and, on the other, by concerns with the escalating cost of institutional care (Chappell and Penning, 1979). This strategy has held particular appeal in rural regions, where cost factors have usually inhibited the development of "intermediate" housing forms catering to the semi-independent elderly and promoted premature institutionalization (Joseph and Fuller, 1991).

Within the broad spectrum of issues associated with the implications of population aging for the provision of in-home health services to the rural elderly, the focus here is on two interrelated themes, one addressing the impact of elderly migration on service demands and the other the question of service coordination. In both instances, the focus is on the Province of Ontario as a representative case, although literature on other Canadian jurisdictions and from outside Canada is drawn upon as appropriate.

Following a consideration of the broad nature and context of the elderly migration and service coordination issues, the emphasis in the remainder of this chapter is on two Ontario case studies, one focusing on the issue of elderly migration and its implications for service provision and the other on the issue of service coordination. The chapter is concluded by an overview of the case studies and a consideration of policy and research priorities.

Provision Issues in Rural Areas

Population Aging in Rural Regions

In discussing the nature and implications of population aging in rural communities, a distinction must be made between the "congregation" and the "concentration" of the elderly. Congregation considers the absolute spatial distribution of the elderly without reference to the remainder of the population; in other words, "where are the elderly?" The number of elderly as a proportion of the total population in a community is a question of relative concentration (Hall et al., 1986). The congregational dimension of spatial distribution is important because it captures the changing location of target populations for seniors programs. In contrast, as concentration of the elderly increases, a shift in the pattern of service needs may occur, such that there is an expansion of demands for special programs targeted to the elderly and a contraction of demands for services and facilities used by younger age groups (Hare and Hollis, 1983; Lee, 1980; Longino and Biggar, 1982).

In Canada, as in other developed countries, it is the relative concentration of elderly persons in rural communities that has drawn attention (Joseph and Fuller, 1991); indeed, a good case can be made for considering relative concentration of elderly as a preeminent indicator of rurality. In Ontario, many rural communities have had concentrations of elderly exceeding 30 percent for a decade or more (Ontario Advisory Council on Senior Citizens, 1980), which exceeds the projected proportion for Canada as a whole when the aging process peaks in 2031 (Stone and Fletcher, 1986). Indeed, on the average, small settlements (1,000 to 2,499 people) in Canada had 13.5 percent of their population over the age of sixty-five in 1981 in comparison with 9.7 percent for the country as a whole, and housed a disproportionate share of those over eighty: 3.1 percent compared to the national average of 1.9 percent (Health and Welfare Canada, 1983).

This is not to say, of course, that congregation levels are not important. Indeed, they are important in their own right in that increasing numbers of elderly persons represent the engine of demand for health services (Roos, 1989), but also because congregation and concentration are demographically interrelated. Migration of elderly persons represents an important focus within this interrelationship and promotes considerable variation in regional demographic structures (Rosenberg et al., 1989) and among communities in the same region (Joseph and Fuller, 1991).

Migration and Population Aging

Population structures are the cumulative record of past patterns of fertility, longevity, and migration. (See chapter 4 for more detail on rural demographic structures and changes.) Within individual countries, migration is usually the most important and volatile source of variation in regional population structures (Bohland and Rowles, 1988). By adding to the numbers of those who have aged in place, in-migration of the elderly can lead to a greater (absolute) congregation of the elderly in a region. If the size of younger cohorts remains the same, or decreases through out-migration, an increase in (relative) concentration will also occur (Hall et al., 1986).

Concentration of the elderly in rural regions has been driven at different times and in different places by various combinations of aging in place and migration. Of particular interest here is the in-migration of the elderly. Although older persons as a group are residentially and locationally more stable than younger cohorts (Struyk and Soldo, 1980), notable peaks in residential relocation and migration occur at retirement age and again after age seventy-five (Wiseman, 1980; Grundy, 1987). Northcott (1988) estimates that overall about 10 percent of Canada's elderly population moves each year. Of particular significance is that at all scales, from local residential moves to long-distance migration, elderly population movement displays a greater degree of locational specificity than that encountered in the movement of the nonelderly (Crown, 1988; Wiseman and Roseman, 1979). In North America, rural regions, particularly those with the sort of natural and cultural amenities usually associated with recreation and tourism, have emerged as an important attractive force in the migration universe of the older population (Fournier et al., 1988).

In Ontario, and in most other North American jurisdictions for that matter, data on migration to or (especially) within rural regions are not comprehensive. Thus, although we know that settlements with populations between 1,000 and 5,000, found most commonly in rural regions, appear to be favored destinations for older migrants (Dahms, 1987; Hodge, 1987) and that a large number of rural service communities of all sizes are emerging as important locations of elderly population (Martin Matthews and Vanden Heuvel, 1987; Simpson, 1984), we do not know with any degree of certainty the extent to which these geographic concentrations of the elderly are due to in-migration of older persons, as opposed to aging in place and/or the out-migration of younger cohorts. An estimation of the relative contributions of aging in place and in-migration to the aging of a rural county in Ontario (Grey County) and its constituent settlements figures prominently in one of the case studies presented later in this chapter.

Implications of Elderly Migration for Service Provision

Elderly migration has profound implications for destination regions and their constituent communities, especially in terms of the management of expanding demands for human services (Bohland and Rowles, 1988; Rogers and Woodward, 1988). Implications stem on the one hand from the expansion of gross demand as a direct outcome of greater numbers of elderly consumers and, on the other, from the possibility that elderly migrants will make distinctly different demands on service providers (Bohland and Rowles, 1988; Bryant and El-Attar, 1984).

It is widely acknowledged that increasing numbers of elderly residents will inevitably exacerbate long-standing problems associated with the matching of limited service capacity with demands emerging from a scattered rural population (Hodge, 1987; Joseph and Fuller, 1991). In contrast, the role of elderly population composition, namely the mix of aged-in-place and in-migrant persons, in influencing demands for services is less clear (Bohland and Rowles, 1988; Lee, 1980). Rogers and Woodward (1988) and Northcott (1988) suggest that, because they are generally married, healthier, and wealthier, in-migrants are less likely to become dependent on formal health and social support services than are their peers who have aged in place. Yet Grundy (1987) contends that the lack of informal supports built up through kinship and over long years of residence may lead in-migrants to lean more on formal supports. The Grey County case study contributes to this debate by presenting data on the use of in-home services among a sample of aged-in-place and in-migrant residents drawn from two communities.

Service Coordination in Rural Regions

Service coordination is an issue that spans the rural-urban continuum; it challenges agencies, planners, and policy-makers in communities ranging from small rural service centers to metropolitan areas (Chappell et al., 1986). In this generic sense, the majority of concerns with the adequacy of service coordination (and with consequent implications for the welfare of client populations) can be traced to the complex and potentially confusing nature of service organization and to the lack of uniformity in service availability.

In Ontario, as in many North American jurisdictions, a distinction is commonly made between programs and services with a health focus and those of a more "social" nature (Fraser, 1989), with the former administered by the Ministry of Health and the latter by the Ministry of Community and Social Services. At the delivery level, the programs of the two ministries are referred to as Home Care (which includes nursing and rehabilitative therapy, with or without support services like homemaking) and Home Support (which embraces services such as meals-on-wheels, home help, friendly visiting, and transportation), respectively (Fraser and Martin Matthews, 1988). The majority of these services are delivered and consumed in the home, although some services (such as dining clubs and some forms of caregiver respite care) take the elderly person out of the home.

This distinction between in-home health and in-home social support services is often more apparent than real, more administrative than actual (Fraser and Martin Matthews 1988). "Homemaking" under the auspices of the Ministry of Health's Home Care program (involving assistance in, for example, meal preparation, housecleaning, and personal care) is the classic example of overlap, appearing as "home help" in the Ministry of Community and Social Services's Home Support program but offering much the same services to elderly clients. Traditionally, the two programs were differentiated by the fact that homemaking was delivered free under the Home Care program whereas elderly persons in receipt of home help under the Home Support program would usually make a contribution toward its cost. The Ministry of Community and Social Services has recently undermined this distinction by introducing an "integrated homemakers" service available at no charge to frail elderly persons. Perhaps as important (and confusing) from the client perspective is the fact that the same agencies (e.g., the Victorian Order of Nurses or the Red Cross) and personnel are frequently contracted by the two ministries to supply services within a particular community. Thus, it comes as no surprise that elderly persons are often ignorant of the auspices under which they are in receipt of in-home services.

The coordination issue is further complicated by the fact that services have evolved historically in response to local recognition of need. This is especially true of social support services, but a degree of lack of uniformity exists in health-related services too. Fraser and Martin Matthews (1988) point out that this unevenness in provision may be seen as a necessary and desirable response to the heterogeneity of elderly populations, but suggest that it may also reflect the impact of systemic and undesirable constraints. "Rurality," I maintain, is a construct that embraces many of these constraints.

It is widely acknowledged that rurality is a multidimensional construct that defies easy generalization (Martin Matthews and Vanden Heuvel, 1987; Windley and Scheidt, 1988; also see chapter 2 in this volume) and that observed urban-rural or rural-rural differences in phenomenon or process may sometimes be a by-product of the manner in which rurality is conceptualized (Martin

Matthews, 1988). What is not in doubt is that rural communities, however defined, suffer disproportionately from the impacts of poor service coordination; the consequences of service gaps or overlaps are overlain upon the composite effects of a series of geographic and organizational constraints that are endemic to the delivery of services in rural areas (Fraser and Martin Matthews, 1988).

The emphasis here is on the geographic constraints on service delivery. Organizational constraints, stemming either from entrenched community attitudes toward service provision or from contemporary shortages of human resources, are undeniably important, but their effects on service coordination are played out against the backdrop of enveloping geographic constraints. Those responsible for service coordination must face the all-too-familiar challenge of providing services from isolated service centers over large distances to a dispersed client population (Joseph and Bantock, 1984), with the added complication of seasonal impediments to travel (Fraser and Fuller, 1989). This same geographic reality impedes the easy interaction among providers that underlies successful management of client needs in a complex supply environment.

Migration and Service Coordination

The migration and service coordination issues are related in several ways. At the heart of their interconnection is the reality that population distribution (as a fundamental determinant of demand) is a key ingredient in the geography of service delivery and its coordination. The impact of migration on service demands may extend beyond the origin, destination, and magnitude of flows to the differential demands of migrants and nonmigrants (or perhaps even migrants of different origin). Initiatives for the improved coordination of in-home services need to be aware of these and other relationships between migration and service demands. Of particular importance is the known tendency of elderly persons with failing health to move from isolated locations in the countryside to larger villages and towns housing needed services, thereby transferring demands from locations less accessible to providers to those more accessible (Joseph and Fuller, 1991). To what extent would the improved outreach of in-home services to households in isolated locations reduce this tendency and what

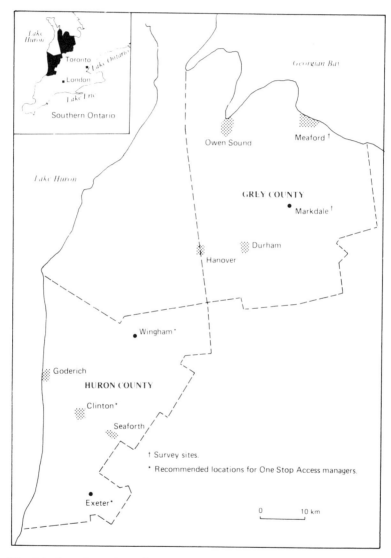

Fig. 5.1. Location of rural senior service use and service coordination studies: Ontario, Canada.

would be the implications, not only for the management of in-home services but also for the continued viability of centralized, facility-based services or assisted-living housing developments?

To facilitate the consideration of these and other questions, se-lected results from two case studies involving the author are pre-sented: the first considers migration and service demands in Grey County, Ontario, and the second the design of the geographic elements of a service coordination strategy for Huron County, Ontario (fig. 5.1). In both cases, social as well as health services delivered to the home are considered; health and social support are taken to be the necessary pillars of continuing independence and their coordination as a fundamental prerequisite for a success-ful strategy for community support of the needy elderly.

The Case Studies

The case studies were carried out in two counties, Grey and Huron, that lie in the rural hinterland of southern Ontario, beyond the commuter zones of the province's larger urban agglomera-tions (fig. 5.1). Evidence presented in recent research by Joseph et al. (1988) on rural population growth in Canada in the 1960s and 1970s and by Rosenberg et al. (1989) on the components of change in the distribution of the elderly population of Ontario between 1976 and 1986 suggests that the two counties are representative of the mainstream of demographic experience in rural Ontario. Grey and Huron do not display the levels of congregation evident in counties in or near the urban heartland skirting the shore of Lake Ontario (Rosenberg et al., 1989), but with relative concentrations of elderly population of 15.6 percent and 15.5 percent, respec-tively, in 1986 (compared to 10.4 percent for the province), they typify the picture of "advanced" population aging painted earlier.

The Grey County Study

The Grey County study is presented in two parts: the first deals with the role of migration in the aging of the county and its constituent settlements, and the second, with the differential con-sumption of in-home services by a representative sample of aged-in-place and in-migrant residents drawn from the town of

Table 5.1. Net Migration Estimates for Grey County (1976–1981)

Age group	Grey County		Towns (n = 4)		Villages (n = 6)		Townships (n = 16)	
	No.	Percentage of 1981 population	No.	Percentage of 1981 population	No.	Percentage of 1981 population	No.	Percentage of 1981 populationn
0–19	15	0.1	18	0.4	50	4.1	125	10.5
20–29	1661	15.2	−88	4.1	−134	−23.2	−841	−17.1
30–44	554	4.1	127	5.1	56	7.8	666	9.7
45–54	140	1.8	39	2.8	−20	−4.8	279	7.2
55–64	430	5.6	113	7.4	22	4.5	228	6.0
65+	567	5.2	443	14.8	116	11.0	−410	−11.3

Note: The estimated number of net migrants is expressed as a percentage of the terminal (1981) population.

Meaford (population 4,380 in 1986) and the village of Markdale (population 1,226 in 1986).

Net migration estimates for the period 1976–1981 were generated from published census data using the procedure outlined by Field (1986), and are summarized for the county and for three settlement categories in table 5.1. The county data indicate a net out-migration of younger persons and a net in-migration of persons in more mature cohorts. Other analysis of the Grey County data has indicated that this situation also existed in each of the five-year periods immediately preceding and following 1976–1981 (Joseph and Cloutier, 1989). Such rates of age-specific in- and out-migration constitute the cumulative demographic platform for the rapid aging of Grey's population in the 1990s and beyond. As a complement to this insight into the role of migration in the aging of Grey, the data for the three settlement categories suggest a considerable degree of age-specific population redistribution within the county. Towns and villages gained elderly population through net in-migration at a rate well in excess of that for the county as a whole, while townships were probably the source of many within-county movers (table 5.1).

Taken as a whole, these demographic data suggest that migration systems operating at the regional level (i.e., bringing people into counties like Grey) must be viewed in conjunction with well-established and predictable patterns of (intraregional) movement between settlements (Joseph and Fuller, 1991). Both types of population mobility have implications for the volume and location of demands on service systems. Consequently, questions related initially to the magnitude and direction of elderly migration, both regional and intraregional, and subsequently to the differential demands of migrants and nonmigrants for services, are ones of considerable importance in any discussion of service provision for the rural elderly. It is to this latter issue of differential demands that attention is now turned.

Two hundred and two randomly selected elderly (aged sixty-five or older) residents of the town of Meaford and the village of Markdale were interviewed in 1987 using a survey instrument based on the conceptualization of the service utilization process set out in Joseph and Fuller (1991) and illustrated in Joseph and Cloutier (1990). In addition to collecting information related to the use or nonuse of a selection of health and social services, the survey elicited information on the background and characteristics of respondents, including their residential history. This approach permits service use patterns to be identified separately for four groups in the sample: nonmovers (referred to earlier as the aged-in-place), local movers, county movers, and distance movers.

Nonmovers are taken to be those who had been resident at the same location for fifteen years or more. This cutoff has been used in other Ontario-based studies of rural aging (Martin Matthews, 1988). Local movers are those who had changed residence within the same community at least once over the fifteen years prior to the survey. County movers are those who had moved to Meaford or Markdale from another location within Grey, and distance movers are those who had relocated from outside the county. This categorization of movers is based on various suggestions in the migration/mobility and service use literatures. For instance, several authors have proposed that local residential mobility differs in composition and motivation from migration (Wiseman and Roseman, 1979; Northcott, 1988), such that local movers are more likely to be moving in response to the stresses produced by age-related increases in physiological and social dependence (Serow, 1988). This difference could well translate into relatively higher rates of service use among local movers. The disaggregation of nonlocal movers into two categories is predicated on the desire to determine whether movers from within Grey (county movers) conform more to the service-seeking behavior of local movers than to that of distance movers. This question obviously has implications for imputing the service demand impacts of disaggregated migration/mobility streams.

The 51.5 percent of the sample who changed residence at least once in the previous fifteen years are spread fairly well across the three mover categories (table 5.2). In terms of tying these data in with the demographic analysis discussed earlier, the proportion of migrants in the sample is estimated to be 36.7 percent (22.3 percent county movers plus 14.4 percent distance movers). This is taken to be a reasonable estimate of the cumulative impact since 1971 of net in-migration of older persons on the age structures of Meaford and Markdale; that is, more than one in three elderly persons currently resident in these communities are likely to be in-migrants.

Table 5.2 presents information on the use of two in-home services, home nursing and homemakers (including home help), regarded as central to the maintenance of the needy elderly in the

Table 5.2. Use of Services by Residential History and Health Status

	Homemaker		Home nursing	
	n	Percent	*n*	Percent
Nonmovers (48.5%)				
"Better Health": *n* = 79 (80.6%)	2	2.5	2	2.5
"Poorer Health": *n* = 19 (19.4%)	3	15.8	4	21.0
Local movers (14.9%)				
"Better Health": *n* = 24 (80.0%)	—	—	1	4.2
"Poorer Health": *n* = 6 (20.0%)	4	66.7	3	50.0
County movers (22.3%)				
"Better Health": *n* = 34 (75.6%)	2	5.9	1	2.9
"Poorer Health": *n* = 11 (24.4%)	1	9.1	2	18.2
Distance movers (14.3%)				
"Better Health": *n* = 21 (72.4%)	2	9.5	2	9.5
"Poorer Health": *n* = 8 (27.6%)	2	25.0	1	12.5

Note: The first set of values for each group is for those giving a self-rating of Excellent, Good, or Very Good Health; the second set is for those giving a self-rating of Fair or Poor Health.

community (Connidis, 1985; Neysmith, 1988). Indeed, earlier analysis of the Grey County data suggests that these two services are very good indicators of service dependence (Joseph and Cloutier, 1990). Use is defined over a two-year time horizon and is cross-tabulated against the perceived health status of respondents by residential history group. In all cases, the small number of users upon which service use rates are based forces a guarded, noninferential interpretation of results.

It is notable that the proportions reporting poorer health are similar in each residential history group, with county movers and distance movers being somewhat more likely to report a less favorable health status. As would be anticipated, use rates are almost universally higher among those reporting poorer health, although this health-based contrast is relatively weaker among county and (especially) distance movers. Indeed, these data suggest that distance movers may be potentially more reliant on formal supports than other movers or those who have aged in place, even when they report better health. Also worthy of note in table 5.2 is the very high level of service dependence among local movers reporting poorer health. Although this factor is not considered here, the survey data suggest that changes in health status (of self or spouse) play an important role in the decision to change residence within the same community (Joseph and Cloutier, 1989), and this may well account for this very high level of service dependency.

On the whole, the data in table 5.2 suggest that movers are a more service-dependent group than nonmovers. However, the nature and extent of dependency (and its probable causality) appear to vary across the three mover groups. Thus, local movers in poorer health stand out as a particularly vulnerable group, a finding that conforms to expectations set out by Wiseman and Roseman (1979) and Serow (1988), among others. At the same time, distance movers in better health appear to be more vulnerable to formal service dependence than healthy nonmovers or fellow (local and county) movers. As suggested by Grundy (1987), this might well reflect the differential availability of informal supports. Indeed, this line of explanation would be consistent with the fact that county movers in better health display an "intermediate" level of dependency relative to healthy local movers (with presumably strong local ties) and distance movers (with presumably limited local ties).

In the Grey County survey the availability of informal supports was assessed via a question on the most important source of assistance available to an individual during periods of illness not requiring hospitalization. The picture of informal supports drawn by these data is a complex one (table 5.3), but amenable to some generalizations. First, and of some concern, is the finding that the incidence of having "no one" to turn to in times of illness (i.e., being forced by necessity to be self-reliant) is usually markedly greater among older respondents. Second, and not surprisingly, the spouse or family represents the frontline of assistance to most respondents in times of illness. However, the relative importance of these two pillars of informal support is completely reversed for the two age groups.

Taking the liberty of extrapolating a temporal, life-cycle trend from these static data, it is speculated that the onset of widowhood with advancing age forces a shift away from the spouse as the main source of informal support. For nonmovers and local and county movers the data suggest that some of the slack may be

Table 5.3. Percent Reporting Various Sources of Assistance
during Periods of Illness, by Residential History and Age

	No one	Self	Spouse	Family	Friends or neighbors	Formal
Nonmovers						
65–74 (*n* = 62)	9.7	9.7	51.6	22.6	4.8	1.6
75+ (*n* = 36)	27.8	5.6	33.3	25.0	5.6	2.7
Local movers						
65–74 (*n* = 15)	13.3	—	46.7	26.7	—	13.3
75+ (*n* = 15)	26.6	—	20.0	40.0	6.7	6.7
County movers						
65–74 (*n* = 25)	8.0	4.0	56.0	24.0	4.0	4.0
75+ (*n* = 20)	—	—	30.0	45.0	—	25.0
Distance movers						
65–74 (*n* = 19)	15.8	—	73.7	10.5	—	—
75+ (*n* = 10)	30.0	10.0	40.0	20.0	—	—

Note: Formal sources of assistance include doctors, nurses, or other medical personnel
and various public agencies.

taken up by family and friends or by agents of the formal support
system. Distance movers, on the other hand, appear more likely
not to have family members to rely upon, to be less tied in to
friends or neighbors or indeed with formal supports, and therefore to be in most danger of having no one to turn to for assistance.
Although it is difficult to relate unambiguously these data on
sources of assistance to service behavior, they are indicative of the
vulnerability of migrants (especially those from a greater distance)
to becoming dependent on formal support services as they age.

The Huron County Study

Following an extensive consultation with seniors groups, service agencies, and other interested parties across the Province of
Ontario, the Office for Senior Citizens' Affairs identified "improvements in access and delivery of services" as a vital prerequisite for the creation of a more effective and affordable system of
health and social services for the elderly (Minister for Senior Citizens' Affairs, 1986, 10). The concept of a "One-Stop Access" case
management system was introduced as part of the resulting

Table 5.4. Assessment of Case Management Location Options

Option category	Key factor	Client/consumer perspective	Case manager perspective	Service provider perspective	System perspective
A. Centralized (single-site OSA)	1. Community visibility and communication	Local disparities in visibility/perception of OSA may lead to decreased use of/access to system.	More time and effort required to publicize/promote their role in outlying locations.	Local providers may become key information/referral agents for clients in the absence of a visible CM. They may not effectively want/be able to fill this role.	Visibility in outlying areas will be dependent on media/information agents and ongoing public relations.
	2. Ease of contact (with clients or providers)	Queuing may be promoted by the need to rationalize CM travel. Frustration over delays in service may result.	Reduced time for assessment as a result of increased travel time.	Delays in assessment or in obtaining relevant client information may frustrate providers or prompt authorization of service before CM assessment is possible.	More time may be spent on travel than on active assessment.
	3. Peer interaction (with providers or other CMs)	N.A.	Increased ability to consult with other CMs. More information sharing and mutual support. Enhanced problem-solving (e.g., for complex cases).	Potentially more removed/isolated from client-service decision-making. Decreased opportunity for informal exchange of information.	Allows for efficient management of CM and global provider resources. Decreases team work among CMs and service providers.
	4. Cost (travel, building)	N.A.	Increased travel to assess clients.	Increased travel time to conference with CM.	Limited building and support staff costs. Decreased operational costs through reduction of duplication, but increased travel costs.

B. Decentralized (multiple-site OSA)	1. Community visibility and communication	High local visibility—promoting understanding, acceptance, and use.	Understanding of CM role enhanced through visibility. Greater awareness of local client needs and priorities and local service resources.	Tendency to assume aspects of CM role (e.g., information agent) diminishes. Reduction in inappropriate information/referral requests.	Locally visible CMs promote OSA.
	2. Ease of contact	Easier physical access to local CM.	Closer proximity to client group, allowing more time for assessment. Greater access to service providers in local area.	Smoother operation of assessment process. Better indication of priorities/goals to providers.	Less time spent on travel increases time for available client assessment and consultation with providers.
	3. Peer interaction	N.A.	Reduced ability to interact with other case managers on an informal basis. Decreased peer support.	Enhanced ability to participate in formal/informal discussions of cases, promoting better teamwork.	More fragmented system for management of CM caseloads.
	4. Cost	N.A.	Reduced travel time, with more time for assessment.	Reduced travel time to case conferences.	Expansion of space, staff needs. Reduced travel costs.

Assumptions: (1) The location of clients and providers is fixed. (2) A telephone contact system and information system will exist regardless of the locational arrangement of the OSA CMs.

Key: CM = case manager, N.A. = not applicable, OSA = One-Stop Access.

Source: Adapted from Gerontology Research Centre and University School of Rural Planning and Development (1988).

policy strategy. A team at the University of Guelph was commissioned by the Office of Senior Citizens' Affairs to develop a pilot model of One-Stop Access for a rural county, Huron (fig. 5.1), and reported in early 1988 (Gerontology Research Centre and University School of Rural Planning and Development, 1988).

The overall objectives of One-Stop Access are far-reaching, involving the localization of important planning and management functions as well as the coordination of support services that are currently the responsibility of two ministries (Health and Community and Social Services) with radically different administrative structures and decision-making hierarchies. Consequently, the development of the pilot model involved, among other things, considerable research and design in the area of service delivery modes and organization, together with consideration of the diverse forms of communication (among clients, providers, and managers) that constitute the sinews of successful service delivery (see Gerontology Research Centre and University School of Rural Planning and Development, 1988). The emphasis here is on the design of the locational arrangement for the case management system, for which the author acted as consultant.

The location of case management question was conceptualized as a centralized-decentralized continuum, with the limits being on one hand the concentration of all case managers at one site and, on the other, the dispersal of n case managers across n sites. Insight into the relative merits of centralization/decentralization was sought through a consideration of four factors believed to be critical to the successful implementation of the One-Stop Access system—(1) community visibility and communication; (2) ease of contact among case managers, clients, and providers; (3) peer interaction; and (4) cost—from the distinct perspectives of clients/consumers, case managers, service providers, and the system as a whole (table 5.4).

Examination of table 5.4 reveals complex trade-offs between the centralized and decentralized scenarios, even within particular evaluation perspectives. For instance, centralization reduces office costs and saves on the costs associated with peer interaction but increases travel costs incurred in client assessment. Consequently, any judgment as to the degree of centralization/decentralization that should be built into the case management system clearly depends on the weight that is attached to the various factors and perspectives.

On the basis of the a priori rationale for One-Stop Access, it was decided that the client perspective should take precedence over all other perspectives (Gerontology Research Centre and University School of Rural Planning and Development, 1988). Indeed, scrutiny of table 5.4 reveals that the case management system works well from the perspectives of case managers and providers almost regardless of the locational configuration of the system. What is more in doubt is whether One-Stop Access would work if it were not visible locally; the extent to which the system is perceived to be readily available and accessible might well be a major determinant of use, and hence success (Gerontology Research Centre and University School of Rural Planning and Development, 1988). Consequently, the design team recommended a partially decentralized system, recognizing the importance of local visibility while acknowledging the many costs associated with decentralization. The recommended locations of case managers were Exeter (south Huron), Clinton (central Huron), and Wingham (north Huron), as shown in fig. 5.1.

Overview

The Case Studies in Retrospect

The development of the One-Stop Access model for Huron County created an awareness of the complex variety of geographic and organizational constraints on the efficient long-term delivery of in-home services to the rural elderly. In particular, the process of designing the location system for case management emphatically reinforced the a priori recognition that the dispersed (and low-density) demand for support services in rural areas constitutes a fundamental and enduring constraint on successful service delivery and effective coordination. The Huron experience also confirmed the almost axiomatic observation that no two rural regions are alike in terms of demand or supply conditions (Coward, 1979; Krout, 1988), in that departures from "model" expectations were frequently noted (Gerontology Research Centre and University School of Rural Planning and Development, 1988).

The Grey County study suggests that for service demands an important part of the variety in rural conditions and experience derives from the migration history of regions and their constituent communities. The Grey County data indicate that in-migrant elderly (especially those coming from distant communities) may be more vulnerable to the early onset of service dependence than those who have aged in place. Consequently, service providers and service managers need to be especially mindful of the potential problems of persons aging in relative isolation from family and friendship networks. This is not to say that a strong net in-migration of elderly persons is necessarily a bad thing for service provision. The growth of demand for services like home nursing and homemaking may produce the economies of scale that have eluded managers of service systems in most rural communities. In-migration, particularly of healthy and socially active younger seniors, may also constitute a vital source of volunteers to assist in the administration and delivery of support services. In the end, the impact of elderly in-migration on in-home service provision will depend on the nature of the service system being affected (Is it efficiently managed? Are resources already overextended?) and the nature of the migration flow (How old are the in-migrants? Are destinations concentrated or dispersed?).

The importance of the age distribution of in-migrants for service provision is almost self-evident and featured extensively in the analysis of the Grey County data reported earlier. Equally important, though, and heavily laden with implications for effective service coordination and delivery, is the degree to which migrants settle in the countryside or in nucleated rural communities. Residence in larger nucleated communities in particular would place migrants in close proximity to services that might eventually be needed, while residence in the countryside (or perhaps even in smaller, unserviced nucleated communities) might further strain already extended agency personnel and travel budgets. In this context a subsidiary comment needs to be made concerning planned retirement communities, of which there are an increasing number in rural Ontario (Ministry of Municipal Affairs, 1986). Planned retirement communities produce a predictable geographic concentration of potential clients for service agencies and, depending upon the degree to which the community accommodates aging, they may reduce demands for in-home services by providing a housing environment more in tune with the needs of residents. Thus, policy on planned communities, and on other aging-related issues for that matter, will influence the future of in-home services.

The Future of In-Home Services

The expansion of in-home services continues to be a central pillar of social policy on aging in the Province of Ontario. It is notable, though, that One-Stop Access has not yet been implemented, even on a trial basis, anywhere in Ontario. Part of the delay stems from an increasing awareness that, in the same way that One-Stop seeks to increase efficiency through better coordination, One-Stop itself needs to be considered in conjunction with other policy strategies.

The basic question is whether or not in-home health and social services represent the best way of efficiently and effectively meeting the demands of elderly persons in need of assistance. No unequivocal response is possible to such a question, saddled as it is with many implicit "ifs" and "buts." What now seems clear, however, is that the expansion of in-home services will not reduce demands (and associated costs) for physician- and hospital-based services. That anyway is the indication from studies in Manitoba (Roos, 1989), a province that has a longer history of comprehensive in-home support for seniors than does Ontario. Another cost-related question concerns the viability of existing or planned housing-based programs in small communities in which the potential demand for accommodation is effectively diminished by the attractiveness of an intervening opportunity, in-home services. The real issue here may in fact be one of social engineering.

The traditional view is that service providers, especially those involved in the provision of in-home services, respond to client needs. The reality is typically more complex, with service managers having to decide who should receive service and when service should be withdrawn and a residential move (possibly into an assisted-housing environment or an institution) encouraged (Joseph and Fuller, 1991). There is always the danger that the overly generous provision of in-home services will make "hanging on" in the family home too inviting, and thereby postpone the stress of moving to a time when the individual concerned is less able to cope. Moreover, service providers will always operate with limited budgets. Should scarce resources be expended on those who can only be maintained in their homes through extraordinary efforts and expenditures? Decisions on issues like these will affect the geography of aging in rural regions by either facilitating the decentralization of elderly population throughout the countryside or encouraging its centralization in service-rich (at least by rural standards) nucleated communities.

Many research opportunities exist in the area of in-home service provision. Rather than outlining specific themes that may be valuable to address, I would like to make a personal plea for a broad approach. Although a valuable enterprise in itself, examination of specific issues in specific locations needs to be cast against the backdrop of a complex rural reality and an interdependent policy environment. There are no policy strategies that will work equally well in all regions or be played out in isolation from other, equally well-founded, initiatives.

Chapter 6

Studying Service Provision for the Disabled
Theoretical and Practical Issues

MARK W. ROSENBERG

AND ERIC G. MOORE

The question "who is disabled" could easily be rephrased to ask "who is not disabled?" For many, the disabled are only those whose disabilities are *measurable*. The disabled are the child in a wheelchair, the middle-aged woman standing on a street corner screaming at her own demons, or the elderly blind man walking with his white cane. But disabilities are not necessarily visible, permanent, or defined in the same way by different people or in different places. There are many people who have hearing, seeing, mobility, and agility difficulties; many who are alcohol- or drug-dependent; and many who have mental problems who refuse to recognize or acknowledge their disabilities, and whose disabilities are not recognized or acknowledged by their parents, children, teachers, friends, fellow workers, or even family physicians. Some disabilities are short-term, others become more severe with time or are recurring. In one setting, a child having difficulties at school might be diagnosed as dyslexic. In another setting, the attitude might be that the child is "just a little slow." It is this complex mixture of measurement, definition, attitudes, and context that makes the discussion of the provision of services for the disabled so difficult.

Beyond these issues, people responsible for health care and social service delivery in rural areas face the additional problems posed by the small number of disabled persons, their geographic dispersion, and the constrained financial resources of local governments because of the generally lower incomes found in rural areas and the limited amount of taxable property. (Indeed, many urban areas are also faced with similarly limited funds, albeit for different reasons.)

Geographers, planners, and regional scientists have already made substantial contributions to the general discussion of service delivery in rural North America (see, for example, Lassey, 1977; Massam and Askew, 1984; Smit and Joseph, 1984; Wolfe, 1984). They have also made substantial contributions to the literature on the deinstitutionalization process and the failure of communities to provide effective integrative services and small-scale facilities for the mentally disabled in urban areas (see, for example, Dear and Taylor, 1982; Dear and Wolch, 1987; Smith, 1988). The study of the disabled and their access to health care and social services in rural North America remains, however, a relatively uncharted area for geographers, planners, and regional scientists.

In this chapter, we address these issues within the framework of four themes: defining and measuring disability, the rights of the disabled, service alternatives, and linking service delivery and the rural disabled. Our focus for this discussion is research that examines these issues within a North American setting. What will become obvious to the reader as he or she follows our discussion is that there are many unresolved issues for which the disabled, physicians, nurses, therapists, and many others will need to join with geographers, planners, and regional and other social scientists to seek the answers in cases in which we can only identify the questions. To this end, our chapter can be read as a framework for further research, and in our conclusion we suggest some areas of study in which geographers, planners, and regional scientists could contribute to research on the disabled in rural North America. We begin, however, by asking "what is the scope of disability in the United States and Canada?"

The Scope of Disability in the United States and Canada

The scope of disability in the United States and Canada is obviously contingent upon how one defines disability. Although there are various accepted methods for defining some disabilities, there are also weaknesses to these definitions and disagreements about what is and what is not a disability. Leaving these issues aside for the moment, in this section we review some *crude* measures of the scope of disability in the United States and Canada, recognizing that some of the differences are a function of the methodological and definitional issues discussed in the next section and that some are a function of the size of the populations of the two countries.

In the United States, Fine and Asch (1988, 5) list various estimates of the size of the disabled population:

> In 1980 Bowe estimated the total population of people with disabilities in the United States to be 36 million, or perhaps 15% of the nation's people. In 1986 ("Census Study"), the *New York Times* reported some 37 million people over 15 years of age with disabling conditions. . . .
>
> The nation's population includes some 10% of school-aged children classified as handicapped for the purposes of receipt of special educational services; . . . somewhere between 9 and 17% of those between 16 and 64 years of age report disabilities that influence their employment situation (Haber & McNeil, 1983); nearly half of those over 65 indicate having one or more disabilities that interfere with their life activities or are regarded by others as doing so (DeJong and Lifchez, 1983).

The figures for Canada provided by the 1986 Health and Activity Limitation Survey (Statistics Canada, 1988) are very comparable. Just over three million individuals or 13.2 percent of the population indicated some level of disability that resulted in limitation of activity. Just over 5 percent of school-aged children were disabled, 5.7 percent of those aged fifteen to thirty-four, 15.7 percent of those aged thirty-five to sixty-four, and 45.5 percent of those over sixty-five. The age structure of disability is very clear, as is indicated in fig. 6.1, which provides age- and sex-specific estimates of total disability for the Province of Ontario; this profile mirrors the pattern for Canada as a whole (Moore et al., 1989).

A second set of measures provides some sense of the scope of long-term disability. In the United States, in 1980 an indication of the size of the long-term disabled population were the 1,426,000 persons resident in homes for the aged and dependent, the 255,000 persons in mental hospitals and residential treatment centers, the 8,000 persons in tuberculosis hospitals, the 61,000 persons in chronic disease hospitals (excluding tuberculosis and mental hospitals), the 149,000 persons in homes and schools for the mentally handicapped, and the 27,000 persons in homes and schools for the

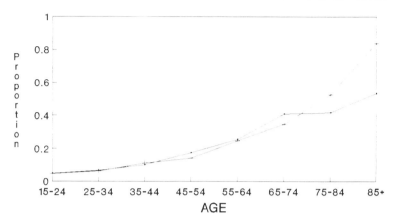

Fig. 6.1. Disability rates for Ontario by age and sex (1986). *Key:* • = male,
+ = female.
Source: Health and Activity Limitation Survey 1986 (1986).

physically handicapped (U.S. Department of Commerce, Bureau
of the Census, 1988, 52).

Although there is some overlap with the preceding data, in 1980
the resident population in all types of hospitals and nursing home
facilities was 2,427,000 (U.S. Department of Commerce, Bureau of the
Census, 1988, 97). With deinstitutionalization, by 1985 the total residential population in hospitals had dropped to 900,000 (U.S. Department of Commerce, Bureau of the Census, 1988, 97). This included
714,000 residents in general hospitals, 143,000 in psychiatric hospitals, 11,000 in chronic care hospitals, and 1,000 in tuberculosis hospitals (U.S. Department of Commerce, Bureau of the Census, 1988, 97).
In addition, 1,553,000 persons were resident in nursing homes in 1986
(U.S. Department of Commerce, Bureau of the Census, 1988, 97).

Although we do not have such detailed data for Canada, the
overall picture is one of slightly higher levels of institutionalization, particularly among the elderly. Overall there were an estimated 247,000 disabled individuals in institutions, with 195,000 of
these being over age sixty-five (Statistics Canada, 1988). Forbes et
al. (1987) reported that about 6.7 percent of the population over
sixty-five in 1981 resided in nursing homes and institutions while
another 0.8 percent were living in hospitals, rates that are somewhat higher than the 6.3 percent reported for the United States
(Gross and Schwenger, 1981).

A third set of measures that provides some perspective on disability in the two countries shows some of the ways in which disability translates into various expenditures. Taking only those categories for which transfer payments can be directly attributed to disability, in the United States, in 1985, federal and state social insurance and related programs paid out approximately $53.1 billion (U.S. Department of Commerce, Bureau of the Census, 1988, 338). In addition, through supplemental security income and public assistance, the blind received $272 million in payments, the disabled received $7.8 billion, and the permanently and totally disabled received $10 million in 1985 (U.S. Department of Commerce, Bureau of the Census, 1988, 353).

In Canada, under the Canada Pension Plan (CPP) and Quebec Pension Plan (QPP), net benefit expenditures for disability pensions were $751.8 million for the 1985 fiscal year (Statistics Canada, 1987, 6-18). In addition, within the federal social security system, $672.0 million was expended for veteran disability and dependent pensioners; out of CPP and QPP funds, $190.9 million was expended on orphans and dependent children of disabled pensioners; Canadian Assistance Plan homes for special care received $798.2 million; and vocational rehabilitation of disabled persons received $199.6 million in 1985 (Statistics Canada, 1987, 6-19). Provincial governments spent $871.2 million on workers' compensation for permanent disability, $1.2 billion on workers' compensation for temporary disability, and $445.9 million for workers' compensation medical aid in 1985 (Statistics Canada, 1987, 6-19).

Although expenditure comparisons are difficult between the two countries because there are many programs in which the disabled receive benefits in financial terms or in services not accounted for in the above data, and because program definitions and eligibility in the two countries may vary significantly, in 1985 dollars, making no allowances for exchange rates, the per capita amounts spent are very similar. In the United States, the total of the above payments is approximately $61.1 billion. Taking the 1985 population of 239.3 million and multiplying by Bowe's (1980) estimate that 15 percent of the population have a disability, the per capita expenditure is approximately $1,703. In Canada, the total of the above payments is approximately $5.1 billion. Taking the 1985 population of 25.3 million and multiplying by the Health and Activity Limitation Survey's estimate that 13.2 percent of the population have a disability, the per capita expenditure is approximately $1,527.

Defining and Measuring Disability

Defining and measuring disability is a complex issue. Distinctions can be made on the basis of whether a disability is physical or mental; whether it is visible or not visible; whether its genesis is through disease, injury, or behavior; and whether a person has single or multiple disabilities. Even these distinctions do, however, have their ambiguities. Most physical disabilities are visible, but chronic back pains, hearing loss, and dyslexia, just to mention a few, are not visible. Although alcoholism and some drug dependencies can lead to physical addictions, they are generally considered mental disabilities, with their origins rooted in people's individual behaviors and the environments in which they live.

Regardless of how one constructs a typology of disabilities, however, three metrics are generally employed to measure them: *functional limitation* or the ability to carry out daily activities, *severity* or the intensity of a functional limitation, and *chronicity* or the length of time one is functionally limited. Having a limp or being confined to a wheelchair are functional limitations. On a perceptual scale of severity, the limp would be assessed as a minor disability, whereas confinement to a wheelchair would be assessed as a severe disability. A limp, however, may be a permanent disability and confinement to a wheelchair may only be for a period of months.

To determine whether an individual or an institution will receive financial support from government or indeed private sources, legal definitions are employed, predicated on a medical-biological framework using clinical methods for measurement. In essence, the definitions of disability are those that can be clearly observed and assessed in a clinical setting. In addition, for adults, incorporated into the definitions is the determination of incapability to perform gainful *labor* over a period of time.

One example of how legal definitions incorporate a medical-biological approach into the measurement of disability can be found in the U.S. Education for All Handicapped Children Act of 1975 (P.L. 94-142), in which handicapped children are defined "as those evaluated as being mentally retarded, hard of hearing, deaf, speech impaired, visually handicapped, seriously emotionally disturbed, orthopedically impaired, other health impaired, deaf-blind, multihandicapped, or as having specific learning disabilities" (Scotch 1988, 167). A second example is the specified lists of injuries, diseases and mental disorders in workers' compensation legislation in the two countries. Whether a worker's trauma falls into a specified category is determined by boards or commissions through evidence given by physicians, hospitals, agencies or institutions (see Burkhauser et al., 1982, 106–113; Ison, 1983, 15–17).

Beyond the issue of what injuries, diseases, or disorders should comprise a list of disabilities, Weaver (1986, 29–30) indirectly shows just how subjective assessments can be within a legal framework based on medical-biological definitions. Beginning in 1980, the Social Security Administration (SSA) reviewed the eligibility of individuals receiving Social Security Disability Insurance (SSDI), resulting in 480,000 being declared ineligible. Weaver writes:

> In the ensuing uproar, the entire governing structure of the SSDI program was challenged. Between the actions of administrative law judges (ALJs) and federal judges, SSA's decisions to terminate benefits were reversed in over 200,000 cases. The states—entrusted to administer SSDI—stopped abiding by federal laws and rules, sometimes halting reviews, and sometimes conducting reviews under self-styled eligibility criteria. And the courts, in a series of decisions, ruled against the secretary of the Department of Health and Human Services on the very rules used for determining eligibility.

A second way in which disability is measured in the United States and Canada is through the use of national surveys. The major purpose of these surveys is to determine the prevalence of disability among the population, the underlying motivation being the need for information for research and policy development.

Specifically, in the United States, within the *National Health Interview Survey* (NHIS) are questions pertaining to "personal and demographic characteristics, illness, injuries, impairments and other health topics" (U.S. Department of Commerce, Bureau of the Census, 1988, 885). The information is collected through detailed interviews of 42,000 households in which one individual provides the information for the entire household. The response rate for the survey is very high (95.7 percent in 1985), although the estimates of sampling error on specific questions may vary considerably (e.g., 3.5 percent for workdays lost by males; 4.7 percent for persons injured at home) (U.S. Department of Commerce, Bureau of the Census, 1988, 886).

There is no equivalent to the NHIS in Canada. As a result, Canada has no continuous source of information on the prevalence of disability within the Canadian population similar to what exists in the United States. In the 1980s, however, three data sources became available. The first of these is the "Canadian Health and Disability Survey (CHDS) which was conducted in October 1983 and June 1984 as a supplement to the Labour Force Survey" (Moore et al., 1989, 6). A second source is a question asked on activity limitations in the 1986 Census. The third source is the Health and Activity Limitation Survey (HALS). It represents the latest and, most comprehensive attempt to identify Canada's disabled population.

Similar to the NHIS, the HALS is based on a probability sample of personal interviews and has a high response rate (90 percent for the household survey). In other respects, it is obviously different in its methodology, how questions are worded, its scope, and most importantly, its main purpose. Whereas the NHIS's main purpose is to monitor the health status of the population in general, HALS's main purpose is to provide a comprehensive picture of disability, although other related issues can be investigated through it.

Two general methodological problems arise out of the use of surveys to measure physical and mental disabilities. One of these is how respondents interpret the questions for themselves and other members of their families. For example, prior to carrying out the HALS, a field test was performed in which a small but nontrivial number of individuals with mild disabilities was found who had responded "No" to the Census question but indicated that they were functionally limited in the more detailed HALS questionnaire (Moore et al., 1989).

A second problem is the dominance of medical-biological approaches to disability within the surveys. Of these approaches, the one that appears to have gained the widest acceptance is the World Health Organization (WHO) concept of the "continuum of disability," whose three key components are impairment, disability, and handicap, defined as follows:

(1) *Impairment* as any loss or abnormality of psychological, or physiological, or anatomical structure or function;

(2) *Disability* as any restriction or lack (resulting from an impairment) of ability to perform an activity in the manner or within the
range considered normal for a human being;

(3) *Handicap* as a disadvantage for a given individual, resulting
from impairment or a disability, that limits or prevents the fulfill-
ment of a role that is normal (depending on age, sex, and social and
cultural factors) for that individual.

(Patrick, 1989, 3)

Patrick (1989, 4) points out that the underlying assumption of
the WHO definition is its sequential nature, which he also sees as
its underlying weakness because "the boundary between functional limitations and activity restrictions is unclear."

Beyond these methodological problems is the issue of how the
sociology of disability affects both the disabled and the non-
disabled in the interpretation of survey questions and responses.
Fine and Asch (1988, 8–15) suggest five assumptions that need to
be considered in defining and measuring disability. First is the
assumption "that disability is located solely in biology, and thus
disability is accepted uncritically as an independent variable."
Second is the assumption that it is the impairment that always
causes the problems faced by a disabled person. Third is that
disabled persons are "victims." Fourth is "that disability is central
to the disabled person's self-concept, self-definition, social comparisons, and reference groups." Fifth is "that having a disability
is synonymous with needing help and social support." This has
led some social scientists, including Fine and Asch, to look to
deviance and minority group theories as frameworks for understanding the dimensions of disability measured.

Deviance broadly defined is "a departure or variation from the
normative standards of society" (Stroman, 1982, 4), whereas a
broad definition of a minority group is its incorporation of four
key characteristics: "identifiability, differential power, differential
and pejorative treatment and group awareness" (Stroman, 1982,
6). Deviance and minority group theories allow the researcher to
situate the measurement of disability within frameworks of interpretation that go beyond external identification of the disabled to
consider the disabled within a consensus/conflict model of society, the relative power/powerlessness of the disabled, negative

stereotypes and discrimination, self-awareness and self-identity, and patterns of responses of the disabled and their supporters that assume discrimination rather than moral nonconformity (Stroman, 1982, 40).

Using a deviance or minority group theory can, however, lead to a conflation of concepts between groups who are functionally disabled and groups who are discriminated against because of their physical appearances but are not necessarily functionally disabled. For example, in "Physically Impaired Minorities," Part Two of his book, Stroman (1982) includes the physically impaired, the blind, the hearing-impaired, dwarfs and midgets, the facially disfigured, and fat people. All are clearly minority groups who are discriminated against in some respects because of their physical characteristics, but it is debatable whether those as a group who are facially disfigured or are fat are necessarily functionally impaired and thus disabled.

Frailty as opposed to disability also poses definitional and measurement problems. Frailty might be defined as a decline in motor skills resulting from aging, such as the slowing of reflexes or a decline in physical strength. It does not easily fit into the WHO continuum because activities are not restricted nor can performance be considered abnormal. It may take individuals who are frail more time to walk the same distance or they may not be able to carry the same weight of groceries as they did when they were younger, but are they disabled? Frailty also does not easily fit into a deviance/minority group framework. Being frail in old age is usually not considered abnormal nor are the frail generally discriminated against. On the other hand, there are environmental designs and services that create impediments for the frail in much the same way that they do for the disabled.

A methodological and an interpretive dissatisfaction with the medical-biological, minority group, and deviance theory approaches to disability has led yet other researchers to suggest frameworks for investigating the disabled and the meaning of disability within societal contexts. Their suggestions include the use of cross-cultural and historical perspectives (Felton and Shinn, 1981; Scheer and Groce, 1988; Simmons, 1982), political systems models (Castellani, 1987), "critical theory" (Dear, 1981; Ferguson, 1987; Foucault, 1989), sociopolitical approaches (Hahn, 1988, 1989) and feminist perspectives (Todd, 1984). In a sense, these suggestions reflect the changes taking place in the social sciences in general, and in the attitudes among social scientists to the study of the disabled in the 1980s. They are a call to researchers to collect information on the *context* and the *environment* in which disability exists.

The more general issue is, however, that the strategies we choose to interact with the disabled population at a public policy level are very much influenced by our conceptual models of disability. Whereas a variety of theoretical perspectives may signify intellectual ferment, they provide little solace to those seeking to make real decisions concerning the allocation of resources.

The "Rights" of the Disabled

Yet another issue that needs to be considered in research on the disabled is the differences in legal rights that exist between jurisdictions and their consequences for individual welfare. Until the beginning of the nineteenth century, support and treatment of the disabled was mainly a private matter in the United States and Canada. In the early part of the nineteenth century, however, there was growing concern to get the insane, the destitute, and criminals off the streets. In the United States, this led to the creation of asylums for the insane, almshouses for the poor, and penitentiaries for criminals (Felton and Shin, 1981). In upper Canada (now Ontario), it led to the creation of an asylum in Toronto as well as a provincial penitentiary and county prisons (Simmons, 1982, 6).

From these beginnings until the end of the 1950s in both countries, legislation in the areas of education, social security, and workers' compensation for the disabled may be viewed as reactions to the unceasing efforts of the disabled and their supporters and the impacts of major events (see Coudroglou and Poole, 1984, 119–127; Statistics Canada, 1987, 6–7; Ison, 1983). For example, the end of World War I led the federal governments of both countries to enact legislation to help disabled veterans support themselves, either through pensions or as an outcome of rehabilitation programs [e.g., the U.S. Vocational Rehabilitation Act (P.L. 65-178), the Canadian Pension Act of 1918, and the Soldiers' Settlement Act of 1918]. In the 1960s, however, a major divergence occurred in the paths taken by the two countries to establish rights for the disabled.

In the United States, with the passage of the Civil Rights Act of 1964 (P.L. 88-352), which included provisions for "nondiscrimination in Federally assisted programs, and equal employment opportunity" (Coudroglou and Poole, 1984, 121), the disabled and their supporters found a new mechanism, the federal courts, to challenge various state actions that discriminated against the disabled. Castellani (1987) cites *Wyatt v. Stickney* (1972), *The New York State Association for Retarded Children Inc. v. Rockefeller* (1972), *Halderman v. Pennhurst State School and Hospital* (1978), and *The Pennsylvania Association for Retarded Children v. The Commonwealth of Pennsylvania* (1972) as the four precedent-setting cases that laid the foundations for the disabled to gain "the right to treatment," "the right to alternatives to institutionalization," "deinstitutionalization," and "the right to education" in regular schools, respectively.

At about the same time as these court decisions, pressure in Congress led to enactment of Section 504 of the Rehabilitation Act of 1973 (P.L. 93-112) and the Education for All Handicapped Children Act of 1975 (P.L. 94-142), establishing "disabled people as a class to be protected from discrimination by federal law," and making "it illegal to exclude them from publicly supported programs and activities" (Scotch, 1988, 167).

The centrality of these pieces of legislation in affecting subsequent legislation in other areas has been noted by various authors (Castellani, 1987; Lewis, 1985; Scotch, 1988). One example is that, in the Surface Transportation Act of 1982 and the Surface Transportation Assistance Act of 1984, Section 317(c), Section 504 of the Rehabilitation Act is used as the basis for specifying public transit options for the disabled and the elderly (Lewis, 1985, 29–30).

In Canada, in the 1960s and 1970s, it is difficult to chart changes in legislation that affected the rights of the disabled because much of the legislation falls within the constitutional responsibilities of the provinces for the delivery of education, health, and social services. Even though the federal government passed a Bill of Rights in 1960 and the Canadian Human Rights Act, creating a Human Rights Commission, in 1977, it was difficult for the disabled to achieve equality because of the legal loopholes within the act and the commission's administrative structure (Parliamentary Committee on Equality of Rights, 1985, 85–86).

This situation changed *in theory* with the passage of the Constitution Act and the attached Charter of Rights and Freedom in

1982. In the charter, equality rights are explicitly granted to the physically and mentally disabled under Section 15(1). *In theory* must be emphasized, however, because of Section 33(1) of the charter, which allows Parliament or provincial legislatures to override Sections 2 and 7–15. While it is unlikely that either the federal government or a provincial government would use the override clause with regard to the rights of the disabled, the very fact that there is the potential to use it means that such an eventuality cannot be dismissed.

Although the federal government, through the Human Rights Commission and other federal departments (e.g., Transport Canada's National Policy on Transportation of the Disabled, the Department of the Secretary of State's Secretariat for the Status of the Disabled), has moved to eliminate physical obstacles in federal transportation facilities and buildings and to encourage more employment of the disabled in government departments and crown corporations, it is likely that the disabled will seek increasingly to use the courts and tribunals, citing the charter in the future (Parliamentary Committee on Equality of Rights, 1985, 82).

In one court decision already, *Huck v. Canadian Odeon Theatres* (Court of Appeal of Saskatchewan, March 1985), using provincial human rights legislation, the court found, in favor of Huck, that "disabled people are entitled to special treatment if that is what is required to produce genuine equality" in access to public services and facilities (Parliamentary Committee on Equality of Rights, 1985, 76).

If this decision does indeed become the basis for a principle of equality of rights for the disabled in Canada, it will represent a subtly different approach than the one that has served as the underpinning for legal decisions in the United States, the normalization principle. Castellani (1987, 14, citing Lakin and Bruininks, 1985, 11) defines the concept as follows: "This standard [normalization] dictates that the residential, employment, and social and recreational conditions of the individual must be close to the cultural norm for a person of that age as the extent of the individual's disability reasonably allows."

To illustrate this difference consider public transit. Under the normalization principle, a disabled adult who needs walking devices could argue that city buses should be equipped with lifts or lowered steps, so that he or she receives *normal* transit services— services that are the same as those received by everyone else. In

Canada, under the *equal but special* service provision, a transit operator could offer a paratransit service and not be obliged to retrofit all city buses.

The importance of achieving equality of rights for the disabled through the courts and legislative bills should not be discounted. However, the control of the states and provinces over how services are delivered and the importance of local authorities in the actual delivery process mean that the potential for discrimination against the disabled and for interjurisdictional inequalities will remain a reality.

Service Alternatives

Historically, service alternatives for the disabled population have been organized between isolated residential settings and special schools at one end of a continuum and community settings and the public school system at the other end of the continuum. However, the swing since the beginning of the 1970s has been toward the *integration* of the disabled into the community, the public school system, and, most recently, the workplace.

In the United States and Canada, the trend toward deinstitutionalization can most clearly be seen for the mentally disabled. In the United States, there were 630,000 people in mental hospitals and residential treatment centers and 175,000 in homes and schools for the mentally handicapped in 1960. In 1980, the number in these institutional settings had declined to 255,000 and 149,000, respectively (U.S. Department of Commerce, Bureau of the Census, 1988, 52). The decline in the number of mentally disabled living in institutional settings was paralleled by the decline in the amount of resources provided. In 1960, there were 722,000 beds in psychiatric hospitals. In 1985, the number of beds had declined to 169,000 (U.S. Department of Commerce, Bureau of the Census, 1988, 98). In Canada, similar trends can be found. "In 1982–83 the number of cases of mental disorders separated from psychiatric hospitals was 36,396, representing a 29 percent decrease over 1971" (Statistics Canada, 1987, 9).

However, the integration of the mentally disabled back into the community has not been so successful (see Dear and Taylor, 1982; Dear and Wolch, 1987), and indirect evidence on the mentally disabled who are elderly suggests that their numbers are increasing in the formal health care system. In the United States, the number of people in nursing and related care facilities grew from 1,076,000 in 1971 to 1,553,000 in 1986 and the number of beds increased from 1,202,000 in 1971 to 1,709,000 in 1986 (U.S. Department of Commerce, Bureau of the Census, 1988, 102). In Canada, people age sixty-five and over "accounted for 9 percent of all hospitalizations and 16 percent of patient days" for mental disorders in general hospitals in 1971. In 1982–1983, they accounted for "18 percent of all hospitalizations and 40 percent of patient days" for mental disorders in general hospitals (Statistics Canada, 1987, 9).

For the physically disabled in general, and especially for the school-age disabled, the processes of deinstitutionalization and integration appear to be more successful. The data that are available come from the United States. They show that, in 1985, 68.4 percent of all physically disabled students under twenty-two years old were attending regular classes, 23.7 percent were attending separate classes, 7.2 percent were attending separate schools and 0.7 percent were served in other settings (U.S. Department of Commerce, Bureau of the Census, 1988, 135).

There is, however, clearly tremendous variation in these data, depending on the type of physical disability, whether the individual has a single disability or multiple disabilities, and in which state the individual resides. For example, 91.1 percent of the speech-impaired population under twenty-two years old attend regular classes, but only 44.9 percent of the hard of hearing and deaf, and 16.5 percent of the multihandicapped, attend regular classes (U.S. Department of Commerce, Bureau of the Census, 1988, 135). Among the various examples of state variation that Biklen (1988, 133) mentions, he shows that, for those labeled retarded, the percentage who attend special schools ranges from 0 percent in Nebraska to 40 percent in Maryland. These variations at the state level raise the question of what variations we might expect within states between urban and rural areas.

Yet another issue that the deinstitutionalization process and integration into the community raise is that, either by choice or necessity, more of the disabled will go through life living with their families. The process of aging, the growing view that the elderly should remain in their homes, and deinstitutionalization mean that care for the disabled elderly is most likely to be in the home, and that the most likely caregiver will be the spouse or the child of the disabled person (see chapter 5 for more on the rural elderly). Although Fischer and Hoffman (1984) use the term "frail elderly," they provide (p. 209) a useful summation of the costs of supporting the elderly disabled at home: "These costs include the depletion of financial resources for the frail elderly and often also for their family caregivers; serious erosions of personal freedom for both the frail elderly and their families; and stress and conflicts in family relationships."

This issue will become even more acute in the early decades of the next century as the percentage of the population sixty-five years of age and over steadily increases, given the much higher rates of disability found among the elderly.

If deinstitutionalization and the integration of the disabled into the community are to be successful, the foregoing discussion suggests that there is the need for a commitment by the community to provide a range of services to the disabled and their family and community supporters. Test (1981) has suggested the types of community services needed for the deinstitutionalized chronically mentally ill. Her suggestions might be adapted as a checklist for community provision of services for all disabled persons. Included in the list are residential services (services to help the disabled find living accommodations within the community); assistance in basic needs ("learning and implementing daily living skills"); crisis intervention services; therapy services; employment, social, and psychological counseling; and services to the family and community supporters of disabled persons (social and psychological support). She also suggests that services be delivered on an individualized basis, that they must be "assertively available," and that there is a need for continuity of care and ongoing rather than time-limited services.

Linking Service Delivery and the Rural Disabled

Health care and social service professionals have a direct and obvious role to play in the identification of disabilities, their assessment, and the provision of most of the services listed by Test. Their ability to do so is, however, severely constrained by their geographic characteristics and those of the disabled in rural communities.

Table 6.1. Number of People Reporting Selected Disabilities in Urban and Rural Places in Ontario (1986)

Disability	Urban number reported	Rate per 100	Rural number reported	Rate per 100
Mobility	563,549	9.4	106,018	9.9
Agility	460,758	7.7	98,127	9.1
Seeing	138,673	2.3	10,985	1.0
Speaking	47,878	0.8	5,188	0.5
Hearing	271,361	4.5	59,159	5.5

Source: Calculated from tables 1–5 in Moore et al. (1989).

The lack of health care practitioners and facilities capable of providing advanced medical care and therapy in rural areas of North America is well documented (Rosenberg, 1983; Rosenblatt, 1981; and chapter 8). Even more critical in rural areas is the lack of physicians in specialties whose services are required in both the assessment and treatment of mental and physical disabilities. For example, Anderson and Rosenberg (1990) note the lack of psychiatrists and orthopedic surgeons in mainly rural northern Ontario.

Compounding the problems of service delivery in rural areas are the small number of disabled, the variety of disabilities, and their geographic dispersion. What little evidence there is shows that the *rates* of various disabilities are similar in urban and rural areas, but the actual number of disabled in rural areas will be relatively small when comparing urban and rural areas overall, and very small within any individual rural community. Table 6.1 illustrates some of these similarities and differences.

Faced with the distributional characteristics of health care delivery personnel and facilities and the disabled previously described, in the short term, health care and social service planners in rural communities must decide whether to centralize all services in one location, locate "packages" of services in key locations, try to disperse all services throughout the jurisdiction, or bring the services to the disabled at home, in the schools, or at their workplaces. Each option has its strengths and weaknesses (see chapter 5). In linking service delivery and the disabled in rural areas, then, a key issue becomes the role of transportation.

In rural areas, it may even be easier than in urban areas to provide transit services to the disabled attending regular schools because in many areas most children attending school are bused. To fit some school buses with a lift or other device to make them accessible on those routes where disabled children live should be possible. Identification, assessment, and therapy could then be carried out by health care and social service professionals using schools as the focus for the delivery system.

For the adult disabled, the provision of transit services to link them to the health and social service delivery system, and indeed other everyday activities, is, however, more problematic because of the complete absence of transit services in many rural areas. Although the number of disabled who need transit services within a particular rural community may be small, the importance of transportation services for the disabled still needs to be stressed. Moore et al. (1989, 15) show that in Ontario over 30,000 disabled persons indicated that they are housebound because of the non-availability of special services, and a further 15,000 who are not housebound say they perceive a need for special transportation services but none are available. Among this latter group, 11,000 live in places where no suitable transit services exist whatsoever.

Where there are no transit operators, local governments or voluntary associations would be the likely candidates to provide paratransit services. They would, however, be faced with the same problems as private operators: small numbers and highly dispersed locations, resulting in a service that would operate infrequently and over relatively long distances, with long travel times making the cost per trip of operating a paratransit vehicle prohibitively expensive.

An alternative that has been tried in some cities in North America has been the use of taxis subsidized by the local government, and such a system might prove viable in rural areas as well, as a method of linking the ambulatory disabled to the health and social service delivery systems at selected locations within a rural area. For the very small segment of the disabled population (mainly among the elderly disabled) who are incapable of leaving their homes, a greater commitment will have to be made by health care and social service professionals to provide in-home services.

In many places in rural North America, in-home services for the disabled are already being provided. The type of services, their quality, the frequency at which they are offered, and eligibility for them are, however, highly variable from jurisdiction to jurisdiction. Brink (1984) indirectly illustrates the variability in types of services by province in her inventory of programs for the elderly living independently in Canada.

Over the long term, with rates of disability increasing dramatically with age (see Moore et al., 1989), and the growing size of the rural elderly population in North America, the failure to provide more in-home services can only lead to a return to the greater use of institutional settings for the provision of health care and social services in a select number of locations in rural communities.

Given the changing climate toward the right to treatment, deinstitutionalization, and alternatives to institutionalization for the disabled discussed in the previous section, in the coming years, health care and social service professionals and local governments alike are going to be increasingly challenged to make services as accessible to the rural disabled as they are to the general population.

The Disabled, Geography, and Rural North America

Using the subheadings of this chapter as a framework, we conclude with some suggestions of where geographers, planners, and regional scientists might contribute to the study of the disabled in rural North America.

Under *scope of disability*, geographers, planners, and regional scientists might employ some of their growing expertise in spatial demography and statistics and geographical information systems to identify the geographic distribution of the disabled by small areas in rural North America. Studies of the *meaning of disability* in rural communities might be examined in the context of the new cultural geography, with its emphasis on ethnography and oral histories (e.g., Cosgrove, 1987; Ley, 1985). The spatial and operating characteristics of existing or proposed services for the disabled could be assessed to determine whether they meet the legal criteria of rights. *Rights* could also be used as the basis for identifying interjurisdictional inequalities and lead to the analysis of why such inequalities exist through the comparison of various jurisdictions. Perhaps the area in which geographers, planners, and regional scientists could contribute most is in the design, implementation, and evaluation of *service alternatives* that *link* the rural disabled to health and social delivery systems. Using concepts from "the geography of public finance" (R. J. Bennett, 1980), the costs and benefits of various spatial configurations of "packages" of services might be assessed within the limits of the abilities of rural local governments to finance them. The role of transportation in service delivery, the spatial distribution of demand for transport services, providing transport to the disabled versus transporting service providers to the disabled, and assessing the need for transport through the analysis of the socioeconomic characteristics of the disabled are topics for which geographers, planners, and regional scientists have already demonstrated expertise in an urban context (e.g., Lewis, 1985; Wachs, 1979) that could be applied in a rural context. The whole issue of the migration of the elderly, who are likely to become increasingly disabled with age, is yet another fundamental question for the design of health care and social service systems in rural environments that has a significant geographic dimension, to the study of which geographers, planners, and regional scientists might contribute their knowledge. Finally, we should be willing to become activists in support of the disabled in their battles to achieve equality.

The preceding list of suggested topics to which geographers, planners, and regional scientists might contribute their expertise is not meant to be inclusive. Nor should the reader gain the impression that some have not already made significant contributions in research and activism in these areas. If geographers, planners, and regional scientists are, however, to shift the disabled, geography, and rural North America from a minor topic of interest to a topic that garners more attention, then the first step must be a commitment by them to make the examination of discrimination against all minority groups a major theme in geography, planning, and regional science.

Chapter 7

An Ecological Perspective on Children's Mental Health in Northern Ontario

G. BRENT HALL, SYDNEY J. PARLOUR,

GEOFFREY B. NELSON, AND

RICHARD T. WALSH

In this chapter we focus on a particular aspect of rural health care, namely children's mental health, in a geographic setting, northern Ontario, that is rich in both its physiographic and human diversity and conspicuous for its remoteness in a Canadian province where economic prosperity and population distribution are highly concentrated in the south.

The issue of children's mental health and the geographic context typify what might reasonably be described as cases of neglect. Rural mental health issues have, at best, received very sporadic attention over the past fifty years in North America. Furthermore, in Canada, mental health services are within the jurisdiction of each province to design and manage. Most Canadian provinces contain vast stretches of sparsely populated land and governments have had to devise means of servicing their rural populations. One province, British Columbia, has been a leader, in conjunction with the federal body Health and Welfare Canada, in documenting the development of its rural mental health services. Yet rural mental health issues in general and particularly those regarding children have not been adequately addressed in Canada and only now are decision-makers realizing that urban models and approaches to mental health services are not directly transferable to rural and remote areas (Abrahamson, 1980).

Children's mental health services in Ontario have until recently tended to fall between the cracks of two provincial ministries, those of Health and of Community and Social Services (MCSS), with two very different operating philosophies. In addition, northern Ontario, although a major source of Ontario's resource-based wealth, falls behind the rest of the province on almost every socioeconomic indicator. Recognition of health care problems in this area and implementation of policy and programs to overcome health inequities remain among the major health challenges in this province.

Our objective here is to present the problem of children's mental health care in northern Ontario within a general conceptual framework that allows this issue to be viewed and understood from the perspective of the individual and his or her physical, socioeconomic, and human environment. The framework adopts an ecological perspective as its rationale. Within this, we identify three major dimensions of the social context of children's mental health: (1) the geosocial system, (2) the sociocultural system, and (3) the planning, policy, and service delivery system.

The geosocial system refers to the patterning of socioeconomic indicators in geographic space. In northern Ontario, important components of the geosocial system consist of the population size, population distribution, and movements in business and employment indicators. The sociocultural system includes the norms, values, and traditions of families, communities, and rural life in general. Moreover, there are sizable indigenous and francophone populations in northern Ontario that require special consideration. The planning, policy, and service delivery system is concerned with formal health, social, and education systems, and with linkages between these and the economic system.

In the sections that follow we review each of these three major dimensions of the social context of children's mental health in northern Ontario. First, the ecological perspective is presented as the basis of our conceptual framework.

The Ecological Perspective

Borrowed from biology, the ecological perspective emphasizes the importance of the interaction of the person with his or her physical, socioeconomic, and human environment. Trickett (1984) has outlined four principles that define this perspective.

Interdependence. The principle of interdependence asserts that the different components of an ecological system are interconnected and that change in one part of the system will lead to change in another part. Moreover, this principle suggests that there are different levels of systems, with smaller systems nested within larger systems. Bronfenbrenner (1977, 1986) has elaborated an ecological framework for child development with four levels of analysis. The first level is the individual child. Although the family is the basic context for child development, the child is also embedded in other small systems, such as schools, daycare, peer groups, and recreation activities. These interdependent small systems constitute the second level, which Bronfenbrenner calls the "mesosystem." The next level does not contain the developing child but affects the child indirectly by impinging upon the small systems in which the child is embedded. This third level, the "exosystem," includes the parents' world of work, parents' social networks, the community, and the strains and support that stem from these sources. The final level is the "macrosystem," which refers to societal norms, values, and institutions, including the cultural, economic, social, educational, legal, and political systems. These overarching social institutions shape the exosystems (work, school, community), which, in turn, have a direct impact on the child's social network of parents, siblings, peers, teachers, and other caregivers. Belsky (1980) has provided a concrete illustration of the utility of the ecological perspective for understanding child abuse. He has shown that economic conditions and social norms about the acceptability of using corporal punishment can affect unemployment and neighborhood life in a way that increases parents' stress and erodes their support. In turn, these conditions lead to abusive parenting, which negatively influences the child's well-being.

Macrosystem changes in population and the economy will have an impact on particular rural and remote communities (exosystem), which will in turn have an effect on families and other primary groups (mesosystem) and children (individual level). In examining northern Ontario, the family and informal networks (mesosystem); the culture of work, school, and leisure settings (exosystem); and rural community culture and lifestyle (macrosystem) are of central importance. Moreover, the availability and accessibility of health, social, and educational services to children at the community level (exosystem) and provincial planning and policy (macrosystem) can serve either to enhance or to erode the mental health of children.

Cycling of resources. This principle calls attention to the distribution and utilization of natural, economic, and human resources in a system. Management, conservation, and recycling of these resources are important for maintaining a balanced ecosystem. Just as natural resources in northern Ontario are exploited with little regard for the physical or human environment, so too can human service workers be "burned out" if they are isolated and unsupported. This principle also recognizes the importance of informal resources in rural environments, such as norms of sharing and helping within social networks and learning to perform many day-to-day functions independently without having to rely on expert help.

Adaptation. This principle asserts that people must cope with and adapt to environmental demands and changes. Successful adaptation is a function of the strengths and resources of the individual and the environment and the stress created by environmental demands and changes. With regard to children's mental health, various factors that place a child at risk for developing mental health problems have been identified, including physical, emotional, and sexual abuse (Wolfe, 1987; Bagley and MacDonald, 1984); peer rejection (Parker and Asher, 1987); marital discord (Emery, 1982); parents' life stress and strains (Stolberg et al., 1987); and economic hardship (Garbarino and Crouter, 1978; Steinberg et al., 1981). On the other hand, several protective factors have also been identified that help children to cope with and withstand various stressors (Rutter, 1987). These include social problem-solving skills (Hymel and Rubin, 1985), positive parenting (Patterson et al., 1989), peer support (Furman and Buhrmeister, 1985), and positive school and neighborhood climates (Rutter et al., 1979; Unger and Wandersman, 1985).

Succession. This principle asserts that people and systems are constantly changing and that child, family, and community development must be viewed with a long-term perspective. Moreover, this principle recognizes the importance of planning for the prevention of individual and community problems, such as the deteriorating mental health of community members. Community problems are rooted in a historical context and "quick-fix" solutions are unlikely to have any long-term impact. Unfortunately, many attempts at planning do not seem to take seriously the need for a long-term perspective.

In emphasizing the interconnection of elements in an ecosystem, the conservation and management of resources, and the processes of adaptation and change, the ecological metaphor provides a framework within which to understand the problems facing children's mental health in rural and remote areas. Moreover, the ecological metaphor has broad applicability, with a potential to cut across disciplinary boundaries and integrate into a unified framework phenomena that are of interest to geographers, sociologists, community psychologists, and planners. In the sections that follow, we use the principles of the ecological perspective to understand children's mental health in the context of the (1) geosocial, (2) sociocultural, and (3) planning, policy, and service delivery contexts of northern Ontario.

The Geosocial Context of Northern Ontario

Geographers have underscored the importance of viewing mental health in its geosocial context. The geosocial context refers to the patterning of socioeconomic indicators in geographic space. For the purposes of this chapter, northern Ontario is defined by the twelve territorial districts north and inclusive of Muskoka and Nipissing to the south (less than two hours north of Toronto), west to the Manitoba border, and east to the Quebec border. This region is coincident with the north regional boundary of the provincial MCSS and the northeast and northwest Ontario District Health Council regions of Cochrane, Manitoulin-Sudbury, Algoma, Kenora, Rainy River, and Thunder Bay, respectively.

Northern Ontario, so defined, covers 90 percent of the province and has 835,000 residents, less than 10 percent of the provincial population (table 7.1). Historically, the economy of this region has been tied to natural resource exploitation of forestry and minerals and is heavily dependent upon the operations of multinational resource-based corporations. Compounding the obvious development obstacles caused by the dispersed settlement pattern are the large distances between the five major regional centers of 40,000

Table 7.1. Demographic Characteristics of Northern Ontario

Location	1986 population	Percentage change, 1981–1986	Area (km^3)	Population density (per km^2)	Proportion of children 0–14 years to total population
Algoma	131,841	−1.3	51,206.90	2.6	23.9
Cochrane	93,712	−3.3	145,618.01	0.6	24.3
Kenora	52,834	−11.1	396,871.08	0.1	25.7
Manitoulin	9,823	−10.7	3,678.92	2.7	22.9
Muskoka	40,235	4.9	403.29	4.4	19.4
Nipissing	79,004	−1.6	18,011.59	3.4	22
Parry Sound	33,828	0.9	10,056.58	1.4	20
Rainy River	22,871	0.3	16,817.14	0.6	23.5
Sudbury District	22,771	−4.8	43,275.06	0.6	27.8
Sudbury Regional Municipality	152,476	−4.6	2,607.02	0.6	22.4
Thunder Bay	155,673	1.1	109,564.22	1.4	21.9
Timiskaming	40,307	−2.4	12,705.39	3.2	22.6
Ontario North	835,375	−2.7	806,732.99	0.98	23.0
Ontario South	8,266,319	6.4	110,000.71	75.58	20.3
Ontario total	9,101,694	5.5	916,733.70	9.9	20.5

Source: Statistics Canada (1986).

residents or more (Thunder Bay, Sault Ste. Marie, Timmins, Sudbury, and North Bay) that comprise 75 percent of the area's population. In contrast, of the forty to fifty single-resource communities in the north that comprise 25 percent of the area's population, over 60 percent have fewer than 2,500 inhabitants. Additionally, northern Ontario is also home to approximately 33,000 status Indians (50 percent of the provincial total) and a significant francophone population (Statistics Canada, 1986).

The problems of single-resource communities are well documented (see special supplement to the *Canadian Journal of Community Mental Health*, 1983, 3[1]: "Psycho-social Impacts of Resource Development in Canada: Research Strategies and Applications"). Such problems include resource depletion and vulnerability to world commodity prices; vulnerability to corporate policy changes and the cyclical nature of resource industries; increasing

rates of unemployment; declining age and sex-specific populations; difficulties of attracting and keeping professionals because
of harsh climates and isolation; social problems associated with
downturns in economic cycles and income loss; and high costs of
living and doing business (Ministry of Mines and Northern Development, 1986). Symptomatic of the uncertainties associated with
these factors is the loss of population from northern Ontario between 1981 and 1986. In general, northern Ontario lost 2.7 percent
of its 1981 population over this period, while some areas, such as
the mining centers of Sudbury and Kenora, lost between 4 and 11
percent of their populations. In contrast, the population of southern Ontario grew by 6.4 percent over the same period and Ontario
as a whole showed similar growth, fueled by expanding opportunities concentrated in the south.

Inspection of socioeconomic indicators evokes southern stereotypes of the north. For example, unemployment in northern Ontario, although somewhat variable from district to district and
from year to year, is generally 50 percent higher than in the south
(Statistics Canada, 1986). There has been some growth in service
sector employment in the north, primarily through decentralization of government departments (both provincial and federal).
However, this has only served to mitigate stagnation and decline
in the primary sector. Approximately 30 percent of the workforce
in northern Ontario is directly involved in primary industries and
over 70 percent of manufacturing jobs are dependent upon resource industries. Economic decline in these highly important
sectors can have significant repercussions in the communities they
support.

The lack of employment opportunity for young people pro-
duces high age-specific net out-migration south in search of employment, leaving behind a population that is aging more rapidly
than the rest of the province and that has a higher proportion of
children relative to total population than the south and Ontario as
a whole (table 7.1). Unemployment trends are directly related to
relatively lower family incomes and a higher incidence of low
income and transfer payments (including unemployment insurance) in northern areas than in the province as a whole.

Taken in context these indicators are suggestive of composite
"stressful life events" that are assumed to be central agents in the
development of mental illnesses (Dohrenwend and Dohrenwend,
1974). Such events have a tendency to cluster at certain points in

the life cycle and are closely tied at the individual level to the condition of the economy at any given point in time (Catalano and Dooley, 1977, 1979). Consequently, regions that are characterized by the stresses of economic cycles such as those mentioned earlier would be expected to experience, in general, more adverse effects of economic uncertainty on the mental health of their residents than economically "healthier" regions.

One of the best-documented influences on reported symptoms of adult psychiatric disorder is the loss of employment (Stokes, 1985). This is differentiated from the inability to find a first job or the unsuccessful return to employment after a voluntary withdrawal from the workforce, both of which have also been shown independently to influence the incidence of mental illness (Gurney, 1980; Catalano, 1979). Of particular concern in this chapter is the effect of economic regression on the mental health status of parents and consequently on the mental health of their children. Research at the individual level consistently reports that job loss and the inability to find work are more common among known child abusers than would be expected by chance (Garbarino and Crouter, 1978; Steinberg et al., 1981; Watkins and Bradbard, 1982). Moreover, three studies (Conger et al., 1984; Elder et al., 1985; Lempers et al., 1989) have used path models to demonstrate that economic hardship is related to high levels of negative parenting (e.g., rejection, inconsistent and harsh discipline) and low levels of positive parenting (e.g., nurturance, warmth, guidance), which, in turn, are related to children's psychological well-being. Taken together, this research points to the ecological interdependence of children's well-being, parents' well-being, local employment conditions, and macroeconomic conditions. Moreover, it is important to note the volatility of these conditions over time.

Given that northern Ontario does not fare as well as southern Ontario in terms of socioeconomic indicators, the ecological perspective and the research reviewed above suggest that there should be higher rates of children's mental health problems in the north than elsewhere. Two sources of data are germane to this hypothesis: (1) the findings of a province-wide epidemiological study of children's mental health and (2) public records of child abuse documented by child welfare services. The study of child mental health reports on the mental health problems of children between the ages of four and sixteen years sampled in 1981 from large urban (population >25,000), small urban (3,000–25,000), and rural (<3,000) communities in each of four MCSS catchment areas, including the north (Boyle et al., 1987; Offord et al., 1987). Prevalence rates of various childhood mental health problems were estimated, based on parent, teacher, and children's ratings on a behavior checklist and clinical assessments. A sophisticated sampling methodology was used, and there was a high participation rate (91 percent). A few of the findings of this study are pertinent here. First, the six-month prevalence rates of one or more disorders was 18.1 percent for the province as a whole and 16.7 percent for northern Ontario. Rates of utilization for mental health and social services were 6.5 percent for the province and 8.7 percent for northern Ontario.

These data do not consistently support the contention that the north should have higher prevalence rates than the south. One reason for this is that this epidemiological study did not sample indigenous people on reservations in northern Ontario. Extremely high prevalence rates of social and mental health problems among adults and children living on reservations have been documented in other research (see E. M. Bennett, 1985, for a review of these data). Moreover, although never accurately enumerated, indigenous people account for at least 4 percent of the population of the north and likely up to 10 percent in all if nonstatus off-reservation Metis are included. Thus, the failure to include indigenous people in the northern portion of the province-wide survey may have led to a significant underestimation of overall prevalence rates in this area. A second point to note is that these data are now almost a decade old and, although results have only recently been published (Boyle et al., 1987), prevalence and service utilization rates are likely to have changed over the intervening period.

The child abuse data, on the other hand, are more current and provide some measure of support for our contention that children in the north are at greater risk of abuse than children in other parts of the province. Official child abuse data refer to the number of instances in which the local child welfare system has investigated a case and determined that neglect or abuse of a child has occurred. Inspection of table 7.2 indicates that rates of abuse declined substantially in the central, southeastern, and southwestern MCSS areas from 1986 to 1988. In contrast, the rate in northern Ontario increased in 1987 and remained very high during all three years. In 1988 the rate in the north was three times higher than that in the central area and substantially higher than that in the

Table 7.2. Rate of Child Abuse per 10,000 Total Population (1986–1988)

	1986				1987				1988			
	N	SW	C	SE	N	SW	C	SE	N	SW	C	SE
Total children 0–14 years	191,100	583,420	716,245	378,735	190,850	584,360	731,910	386,080	169,030	586,680	750,510	393,930
Number of abuse cases	233	725	550	543	311	614	426	441	209	481	301	285
Rate per 1000 total children 0–14	12.2	12.4	7.7	14.3	16.3	10.5	5.8	11.4	12.4	8.2	4.0	7.2

Sources: Canadian Census and Ontario Child Abuse Register.
Note: Child is defined here as newborns to fourteen-year-olds. Population data for 1986 are derived from the Canadian Census for that year; 1987 and 1988 population data are projections based on medium fertility, mortality, and migration.
Key: MCSS catchment areas: N = northern, SW = southwestern, C = central, SE = southeastern.

southwest and southeast. Also during this period the number of children aged birth to fourteen years decreased by 11.5 percent in the north while growth in numbers was experienced in all other areas.

Results of epidemiological research do not adequately address the ecological principles of resource cycling and adaptation, which are likely to play very different roles in rural and remote communities than in urban areas. Extant research has not examined potential differences in the frequency and intensity of stressful life events and daily stressors between rural and small-town communities, and medium-sized and large urban communities. Moreover, the role of resource factors such as the ethic of self-reliance and mutual help, as it applies in rural communities, has not been adequately studied. In the next section, we consider some characteristics of the sociocultural system that we believe are important for understanding children's mental health in northern Ontario.

The Sociocultural Context of Northern Ontario

In this section, we consider some of the norms, values, and traditions of families, communities, and rural life in general that are relevant to an understanding of children's mental health. We begin by describing the cultural heritage of people in northern Ontario, focusing particularly on native people. Then we consider the culture of rural life in a more general sense.

Northern Ontario is arguably as culturally diverse as the cosmopolitan centers of the southern part of the province. A large francophone population, especially in the northern area approaching the Quebec border, and an indigenous Indian population, which has never been accurately enumerated, characterize this region. The indigenous population of the north comprises off- and on-reservation components. The primary groups are Metis, who are the progeny of Indian and European parents, and status Ojibway and Cree. The latter have treaty rights for some bands dating back to 1850 (Patterson, 1972).

Among the indigenous peoples, many groups continue to live on small reservations that come under the jurisdiction of the federal Department of Indian Affairs. For these reservation-based groups, there is jurisdictional confusion between federal and provincial departments and ministries when it comes to the provision of mental health services to children and their families. Though this uncertainty of responsibility for service does not technically exist with those indigenous families living off the reservations, in reality the children's mental health services available in the north rarely effectively reach either group. There is clear cultural reluctance among the indigenous peoples of the area to use conventional children's mental health care services, given negative historical experiences with provincial child welfare agencies. Indeed, even in 1980, when the practice of placing indigenous children in white foster homes was on the decline, the proportion of indigenous children in foster care in Ontario was still several times the average rate (Johnston, 1983).

Of the service access points available in northern Ontario, indigenous children and families most often come into contact with mental health services through the school system, with teachers, principals, and guidance personnel providing the impetus. The lack of culturally relevant mental health services, or, conversely, the need for services that approach the life of an indigenous child and family holistically, is a critical factor in the widening gap between indigenous and other peoples with respect to the utilization of mental health services. Emergent organizations such as the Ontario Metis and Aboriginal Association, headquartered in Sault Ste. Marie, and the Ontario Federation of Indian Friendship Centers, placed throughout the north, are beginning to assert themselves in bringing the cultural and health care needs of on- and off-reservation indigenous peoples to the attention of government. Indeed, by 1981, with provincial government support, eight child welfare agencies and twenty-one bands had agreed to participate in services under local control in which the emphasis was on indigenous family support rather than apprehension and guardianship (Johnston, 1983). A core dimension of indigenous communities is family life revolving around the extended family and village (E. M. Bennett, 1985). It is within this cultural context that traditional cultural values are conveyed. Consequently, contemporary services for both on- and off-reservation communities rely on family support and cultural education as key therapeutic ingredients (McKay, 1987).

An example of the move toward assertion of nontraditional mental health care practice within indigenous communities is the case of the program northwest of Thunder Bay in Sioux Lookout, where some 12,000 native Canadians are spread across twenty-seven reservations. Through this program six reservations in one area have indigenous counselors providing mental health services in Cree and Ojibway languages (Timpson, 1983). Moreover, the program seeks to transfer mental health service delivery by teaching conventional diagnostic and treatment skills modified to suit indigenous culture. This is regarded as an important innovation, as indigenous-European differences in nonverbal communication, for example, render conventional psychotherapy virtually impotent in the treatment of mental illness among these groups (McShane, 1987).

Such cycling of resources within and among indigenous communities, families, and individuals is likely to achieve eventually improved aggregate mental health. Implicit within the sociocultural issues discussed earlier is the recognition that improvement in mental health status is a long-term process that requires both community and economic development that is sensitive to cultural issues and that is directed by native people (E. M. Bennett, 1985).

Another important dimension of the sociocultural context of northern Ontario is the status of francophone communities in the north. French-speaking residents make up 20 percent of the total population of northern Ontario as compared to only 6 percent of the total population of the province. Over 90 percent of the francophones in the north live in the northeastern districts of the region adjoining the province of Quebec. Recent provincial legislation has compelled provincially funded children's mental health agencies located in districts with a francophone population greater than 10 percent to provide their services in both of Canada's official languages, French and English. Six of the twelve northern districts fall into this category and currently are serving children and families in both languages. However, there is evidence that because it is more difficult to recruit qualified francophone mental health professionals to work in the north, these bilingual staff positions remain vacant for longer periods of time, possibly reducing the effectiveness of services available to francophone residents.

Cutting across the sociocultural context of indigenous and francophone residents in northern Ontario is the nature of rural community culture in general and its relation to mental health practice in particular. Characterizations of rural and indeed remote communities drawn from the Canadian literature tend to portray such areas as lacking in cultural opportunities (Abrahamson, 1980) and psychologically isolated (Canadian Association of Schools of Social Work, 1976), yet exhibiting a strong sense of belongingness, community identity, mutual aid and self- suffi- ciency (Zapf, 1985), with strong social controls over individual and community behavior (Canadian Association of Schools of Social Work, 1976). Such characteristics tend to exert very pro- found influences, both positive and negative, on mental health practice. On the positive side, researchers have noted that rural community settings allow for practice of principles of community participation, integration of services, and health promotion and prevention (Bell, 1980). Rural mental health practice in northern Ontario best accommodates professionals who are prepared to "unlearn" urban-oriented misconceptions, prejudices, and falsifi- cations of rural life and to develop sensitivity to and respect for cultural differences, especially as far as indigenous communities are concerned, in the north (Collier, 1984; McKay, 1987).

However, on the negative side, communication and access to services in rural areas are hampered by distance, as well as cul- tural, experiential, and linguistic differences. Mental health staff are required to make significant adjustments to their expectations and patterns of behavior (Abrahamson, 1980). Moreover, agency staff must often assume multiple roles, a situation that can result in personal and professional tension in the workplace. The net effect of these factors is a high rate of "burnout" or job stress (Hargrove, 1982; Freudenberger, 1974; Paine, 1982) among mental health workers and a low rate of staff retention for any length of time.

Knowledge of the difficulties associated with rural practice has had the effect of reducing the pool of prospective urban-trained mental health workers prepared to work in the north to those individuals with a genuine interest or those who cannot find work elsewhere. The provincial government has recognized this prob- lem and the importance of recruitment and employee retention in Ontario in its recent initiative, "Integrated Services for Northern Children" (Ministry of Community and Social Services, North Region, 1988). The effect of this program is, as yet, unclear. How- ever, it is noteworthy in that it recognizes for the first time, at the ministerial level, the need to juxtapose the personal and profes- sional needs of children's mental health workers against the sociocultural complexities that characterize the north. It is hoped that such macrosystem initiatives will serve to improve the quality of service provision and enhance the mental health status of children in affected areas. We now turn our discussion to the planning, policy, and service delivery system.

The Planning, Policy, and Service Delivery Context of Northern Ontario

Prior to 1977, children's mental health services in Ontario were provided by a number of provincial ministries. Rapid growth in the number of programs during the 1960s and 1970s with nobody to oversee and manage these developments produced a serious lack of coordination in planning and service delivery. Major gaps in some services, duplication in others, and no system of accountability were symptoms of a service system out of control (Ministry of Community and Social Services, North Region, 1980).

Partly because of a strong bias toward residential services and partly because the majority of these services were in the urbanized southern part of the province, gaps in service delivery became particularly apparent in the north. Professional resources, funding, and government administration were all concentrated in southern Ontario, leaving the north to fend for itself and remain a virtually unknown entity in terms of service needs. In short, the geosocial focus on all things south was reflected in policy, planning, and service delivery of children's mental health care.

In 1977 the provincial government recognized this problem and took an important step toward remedial action by announcing the formation of the Children's Services Division (CSD) of MCSS. This development was coupled with a statement of intention to establish committees to oversee children's services at the local level. The CSD was created to bring together and consolidate under one jurisdiction all programs for children with special needs across the province. The local committee concept was intended "to increase the responsiveness of children's services to the local community, and to increase involvement of the community in the provision of services" (Ministry of Community and Social Services, North Region, 1980, 21).

Ten broad goals were developed by the CSD to guide the development of the children's services system in Ontario during the

1980s. One of these goals, "to ensure equality of services among local areas and regions, while permitting variation according to local differences" (Ministry of Community and Social Services, North Region, 1980, 31), directly addressed the geosocial disequilibrium in the province and the sociocultural diversity of the north, discussed previously. Moreover, the stated intention of the CSD was to develop techniques and information that would enable it to define more precisely the extent of regional and local disparities in service availability. Their goal was, for the first time, to permit a rational analysis of the allocation of funds on a geographic basis and to attain uniform quality of services and access to a full range of services for all regions of the province, while not replicating all services in all areas. To this end, in 1979 the "Northern Priorities" initiative was announced to provide long-term funding for children's services in northern Ontario. Three million dollars was allocated for a number of short-term projects, while other more successional projects were chosen for funding and local working groups were established to articulate the needs of their communities.

In addition to the innovations of the CSD, MCSS decentralized its own administrative operations in the late 1970s in order to be closer and more sensitive to the needs of distant communities. This momentum has been maintained through the 1980s, culminating in the 1988 position document, "Northern Directions for the Delivery of Services to Special Needs Children and Their Families" (Ministry of Community and Social Services, North Region, 1988). In addition, a further major provincial funding program named "Integrated Services for Northern Children" (ISNC) has been initiated to support the goals in "Northern Directions" and earlier policy statements.

Notable among this recent flurry of administrative activity in the north is the establishment of committees composed of representatives of three provincial ministries: Health, Education, and Community and Social Services. As part of an interministerial fact-finding mission to northern communities, representatives on these committees were confronted directly with the need for francophone and indigenous services and the shortage of professionals in the field of children's mental health. As a result, ISNC has allocated funding to hire an additional 124 professionals and support staff to provide services to children in the underserviced rural areas of northern Ontario. Core resource groups will be formed in six of the larger centers in the north and the underserviced rural and remote areas will be served from these six centers. Each resource group will include up to thirteen professionals from the mental health, health, and education fields, and support staff. Moreover, each group will be linked to the small communities of the north through a network of thirty-nine satellite workers with training in the social services. The satellite workers will be referral agents and case coordinators as well as service deliverers.

In addition to this outreach program, MCSS currently funds fourteen children's mental health centers spread across northern Ontario. The catchment areas for these centers remain problematic, however, for they include communities up to several hours away by car and some accessible only by air. Also, only one psychiatric treatment center is currently available for children, in Sudbury, to serve the entire northern part of the province.

As a basis from which to plan and deliver children's mental health services in the north, the recent initiatives in Ontario are laudable in intent. However, numerous problems remain to be solved. Prominent among the inadequacies is the absence of good-quality data with which caseworkers and the ministry can evaluate their efforts. With the advent of the CSD of MCSS, each children's mental health center in the province was required to submit monthly client statistics to a ministry office in Toronto to be input into the Children's Mental Health Services Information System. This process proved time-consuming, the coding criteria for the system were unclear, and little in the way of useful feedback was provided to the agencies for program planning. As a result this information system was abandoned in the early 1980s.

To date there has been no comprehensive replacement client data system. A February 1986 internal document, "Information Technology Strategic Plan," clearly states that transfer payment agencies, such as children's mental health centers, are not required to collect standardized data for each client. Instead, each children's mental health center is to collect and submit to MCSS its own aggregate client data as part of each center's annual service plan. The service plan is a comprehensive strategic plan that describes in detail each agency's current programs, the expenditures for the past year, an estimate of expenditures for the coming year, and a summary of the agency's plans and upcoming service priorities. From this document each agency and the ministry negotiate the agency's funding for the next fiscal year. Thus, at present, the client data to be gathered within each agency are determined by the agency itself, with respect more to meeting the needs of its service planning process than to any long-term, coordinated goal.

Of equal concern to the data issue at the macrosystem level is the placement of children's mental health services within the mandate of the provincial MCSS. While MCSS emphasizes the "care" model of service delivery in the programs described earlier, the Ministry of Health, which ironically has no mandate for children's mental health services, emphasizes more of a "treatment"-oriented service model.

In his major report on the Ontario mental health care system, Heseltine (1983) noted that it is essential that MCSS and the Ministry of Health come to a clear and formal understanding about their respective responsibilities and that this understanding be communicated to the field level. Among the options noted by Heseltine is that children's mental health centers be established as autonomous community agencies with their own boards to be funded on a program-by-program basis by MCSS and the Ministry of Health as appropriate. Such an arrangement would afford children access to treatment when it is required, in contrast to the present approach, which is essentially to protect the child from treatment for diagnosed illness within the mental health system.

Recommendations in the Graham Report (1988) that outline a plan for mental health in Ontario do little to promote implementation of the service model proposed by Heseltine. While identifying native populations and youth (six- to twenty-four-year-olds) among special target groups, the Graham Report avoids the issue of service planning for children's mental health by merely suggesting, in recommendation 7 (p. 10):

> That the Ministry of Health establish Area Mental Health Advisory Boards. . . . to develop strategies for more detailed investigations and make recommendations on those special target groups such as youth, the elderly, ethnic groups, Natives and other special needs groups *which, due to the limited time frame, have not been explored in sufficient depth in this report.* [emphasis added]

Compounding the avoidance of children's mental health issues, the challenges of mental health delivery in rural and remote areas of Ontario are not adequately addressed in the Graham Report.

The policy, planning, and service delivery issues relevant to children's mental health services in northern Ontario therefore remain problematic despite the numerous programs that have been put in place by MCSS. It is clear that none of the four ecological principles discussed earlier in this chapter has been adequately considered by decision-makers. Understanding the insights afforded by these principles into the geosocial, sociocultural, and planning, policy, and service delivery systems in northern Ontario is essential for enhancing the mental health status of children in this region. If these principles are ignored, planners, policy-makers, and service providers will continue to operate in a reactive mode, responding to crises in children's mental health. If the ecological metaphor and related principles are followed, planners and policy-makers will be able to give serious attention to the need for economic development, community development that builds on the strengths of rural communities, and native self-determination.

Summary and Conclusion

This chapter has discussed children's mental health within northern Ontario, Canada, a region notable for its geosocial and sociocultural differences from the more urbanized southern part of the province. An ecological perspective characterized by the four interrelated principles of interdependence, cycling of resources, adaptation, and succession has been offered as a means by which to gain insights into the complexities of children's mental health in this area. Within the ecological perspective, we have discussed three dimensions of the social context of children's mental health: (1) the geosocial system, (2) the sociocultural system, and (3) the planning, policy, and service delivery system.

Research reviewed suggests that areas, such as northern Ontario, that are characterized by uncertain economic conditions and remoteness are more likely to demonstrate high rates of mental illness among adults than economically healthier areas. Moreover, the expectation that economic hardship for adults will translate into higher rates of child abuse and children's mental illness suggests, in general terms, the existence of more unhealthy home environments for children in such areas than elsewhere. Inspection of Ontario's child abuse register for three recent years confirms this expectation, yet results from a province-wide children's mental health study do not produce the same results. The latter impression of rural-urban similarities in children's mental health in this province may, however, be masked by the failure of the provincial study to include the on-reservation indigenous children of the north in its sample.

Within the complex sociocultural context of northern Ontario, resource cycling and adaptation to adversity are ingrained into local communities. Indigenous peoples of the north have recently become more assertive in their quest for self-determination and self-help in many areas, including mental health care. However, the francophone minority in northeastern Ontario is becoming increasingly isolated, with several northern communities officially declaring themselves unilingual in English. Further research into the sociocultural characteristics of rural and remote communities and their relationship to family well-being and children's mental health is needed.

Programs receptive to the needs of children in northern communities are slowly beginning to emerge, yet breakdowns in the interdependencies between the federal government, the provincial government, and local communities and families tend to hinder effective development of children's mental health services. Recent program initiatives offer some hope for improvement in the future. However, the failure to reconcile ministerial responsibility for children's mental health services between MCSS and the Ministry of Health continues to pose a long-term problem. The point remains that unhealthy current geosocial and sociocultural environments for children do not bode well for their future health status as adults. Further understanding of and correction of the circumstances underlying the existence of mental illness and abuse among children in northern Ontario will assist in sculpting a more positive and nurturing environment for future generations.

PART THREE

SERVICE PROVISION AND POLICY ISSUES

Chapter 8

Accounting for Shortages of Rural Physicians
Push and Pull Factors

RENA J. GORDON, JOEL S. MEISTER,

AND ROBERT G. HUGHES

The varied geographic distribution of physicians results from a multitude of pushes and pulls. The imbalance in the supply of physicians between rural and urban areas is not a new problem in the United States (Roemer, 1948), although in recent years the disparity has become more acute. Declining rural economies, rural hospital closures, the rising cost of malpractice insurance, and changes in the technology of medicine are among the factors cited as reasons for the growing shortage of physicians in many rural areas of the country.

The importance of physicians to the delivery of health care services has generated a considerable multidisciplinary literature on physician supply and distribution. The purpose of this chapter is to put this diverse literature within the context of a push/pull typology, one that is used frequently in migration theory for explaining the reasons people move. In this typology, some factors push physicians away from rural areas while other factors pull physicians toward rural areas and enhance prospects for rural location. A variety of factors may also push or pull physicians away from or into urban centers. These may not correspond to rural pushes and pulls; that is, a factor that pushes physicians away from rural locations may not pull physicians to urban areas.

The views expressed in this chapter are solely those of the authors and official endorsement by the Robert Wood Johnson Foundation, the University of Arizona, or Arizona State University is not intended and should not be inferred.

The push/pull typology is used here in a simplified form as a geographic tool in order to make sense of a complex problem and to help identify and differentiate between microspatial behavior and macrospatial behavior. Microspatial behavior puts emphasis on the individual level, or the reasons particular physicians would or would not choose to practice medicine in a rural area. Included are factors such as family background, location of medical training, and choice of medical specialty. Conversely, macrospatial behavior refers collectively to factors that are beyond the scope of the individual physician yet affect locational choices. Factors from the environment that are transmitted to the individual include medical school curriculum, governmental funding programs, and national immigration policies that control the flow of foreign medical graduates.

The chapter opens with background information on the difference between places of need and places with effective demand and on problems associated with establishing a standard for what constitutes an adequate supply of physicians in rural areas. Next we provide an accounting of specific push/pull factors, followed by a discussion with examples at the individual, community, state, and national scales of analysis. Coverage of policy implications concludes the chapter.

A concept to keep in mind when looking at rural areas lacking physicians is the difference between places of *need* and places with *effective demand*. Need is usually based upon the health status of a population residing at a location; demand considers whether the location is a place where a physician can make a living (Doeksen et al., 1988). Many factors discussed in this chapter relate to the fact that often rural places of need lack effective demand. Locational analysis also tells us that there is a tendency for flows of goods, services, and people to run from places of abundance to areas of effective demand or to destinations with effective pulls (Abler et al., 1971).

A pull exerts a directed force with respect to excess supply somewhere else. To help explain why someone moves from community A to community B, it is important to emphasize the *pull* at B rather than the push at A (Abler et al., 1971, 199). Locational analysts emphasize that the pull of demand is primary and that the push of supply separately is not sufficient to support a movement or an interaction (Haggett, 1965; Pred, 1966). In relating physician location to this concept, the push of an excess supply of physicians from community A will not be sufficient to force movement to community B. The force of effective demand at B is the primary variable, or conversely the force of effective demand at A.

Issues arising from the relationship between the supply of urban and rural physicians begin with the absence of a norm for how many physicians a given geographic area should have. There is no accepted standard or set of standards, although analysts have used a variety of methods to estimate what constitutes an adequate or optimal supply of physicians. In general a method of determining how many physicians there should be is used to generate a standard or requirement, which is often reported as a ratio of physicians to population. These methods include estimating requirements based on professional judgment; estimating requirements based on age, disease, and other characteristics of the population (a "needs-based" approach); and estimating requirements based on the past use of services by the population (a "demand-based" approach) (U.S. Department of Health and Human Services, 1986).

Establishing a standard for how many physicians rural areas should have is further complicated by a number of factors. Medical work is divided among the specialties, with considerable overlap between and among the primary care physicians and some specialists (Aiken et al., 1979). For example, in many rural communities the same medical work is often performed by family practitioners and internists. A rural physician's ability and willingness to care for a patient with a particular diagnosis or perform a procedure may depend on training, local custom, or the availability of another physician with expertise. The overlap in medical work is not limited to physicians; nurse practitioners and physician assistants can perform a large percentage of the tasks that comprise primary medical care. These other health professionals can provide an alternative source of primary care services in rural areas, thereby alleviating the need for a physician.

Another factor that complicates the development of standards for physician supply in rural areas is that the geographic boundaries of markets for medical care services are being expanded. Medical care has been viewed primarily in the context of a local service area, but changes in travel patterns, technology, epidemiology, and insurance may be expanding medical care service areas for selected diagnoses and procedures and for some rural populations. Insurance companies have fostered service regionalization for selected high cost procedures to promote both efficiency and quality. Organized systems of medical care, often physician multispecialty group practices, have transcended local market areas and redefined their market to much broader regions. These changes challenge the routine application of simple physician/population ratios as an adequate measure of physician supply.

Even for the nation as a whole, there is no agreement about what constitutes an adequate physician supply, or what standard could be used to determine if a shortage or surplus existed (Schwartz et al., 1988a,b). Canada also struggles with the problem (Lomas et al., 1985). It is no surprise that agreement about a standard for smaller geographic units has remained elusive.

Despite the lack of a universal standard, the supply of rural physicians has historically been viewed as too low (Kindig and Movassaghi, 1987, 1989). Therefore, policy initiatives at the state and national level that address maldistribution of physicians in rural areas attempt to increase the supply. The objectives of the various programs have been to foster the pushes and pulls that result in more physicians in rural areas and, to a lesser degree, to counteract the pushes and pulls that result in a physician concentration in urban centers.

A Diagrammatic Accounting

The trends in physician distribution result from a multitude of pushes and pulls to and from rural and urban areas. These factors are summarized in tables 8.1 and 8.2. Both tables organize the pushes and pulls into four levels: individual, community, state, and national.

Table 8.1 lists the pulls toward urban centers and pushes away from rural areas that make practicing medicine in rural communities less attractive. These factors tend to enlarge the disparity in physician distribution between urban and rural areas. The table begins with individual factors that affect preference for urban practice location, such as urban origin, professional status and prestige, and higher income potential.

Next are rural community factors that push toward urban location. They include insufficient market area, closure of rural hospitals and/or hospital services such as obstetrics, shortage of other health care professionals, professional isolation, lack of continuing education support, and lack of educational, cultural, and employment opportunities for physicians' families. These factors are common to many rural centers of the country.

Then there are factors at the state or regional level that lend themselves more to urban than rural practice. Many relate to medical education, such as underrepresentation of rural students in medical school(s); lack of rural preceptorships, rotations, and residency training opportunities; emphasis on tertiary and subspecialty medical education, and absence of a rural health office in state or local health departments. State policies on medical malpractice insurance carriers also have an effect.

Last, the table shows national factors that impede physician location in rural areas. They include cutbacks in federal programs, such as the National Health Service Corps (NHSC), Community Health Centers (CHC), Migrant Health Centers (MHC), and Area Health Education Centers (AHEC); weak support from private, religious, and corporate programs; and federal immigration policies that restrict the flow of foreign medical graduates (FMGs).

Table 8.2 lists the rural pulls and urban pushes that increase the attractiveness of rural medical practice. The table starts with individual factors that include gender, family background, and choice of medical specialty. For example, physicians who are female, come from rural backgrounds, and choose primary care specialties are likely candidates for a rural practice.

The table then proceeds to the next level of influence, the community. Is the population of sufficient size to support a solo practitioner? Is the economy healthy and are people able to pay for services by some form of insurance and/or self-pay? Are there sufficient cultural and educational opportunities for one's family? Is a hospital within at least 30 minutes' travel time? Is there support from midlevel providers, and are there opportunities for continuing education? Affirmative answers to these questions would indicate an attractive community in which a physician could locate and maintain a practice. Deteriorating cities and increasing competitiveness in urban medical practice could operate as urban pushes.

At the state or regional level, factors relating to medical education are important. They include medical school admission policies in recruiting students from rural areas, availability of family practice preceptorships, and rural residencies, and primary care emphasis in medical education. The increasing role of state and

Table 8.1. Factors That Decrease Rural Physician Location:
Urban Pulls and Rural Pushes

1. Individual factors
   a. Urban origin of physicians or spouses
   b. Professional status and prestige
   c. Higher income potential in urban areas

2. Community factors
   a. Size and structure of service area population insufficient
   b. Economic weakness of rural areas versus prosperity in urban areas
   c. Lack of diverse cultural and educational opportunities
   d. Loss of rural hospitals or specialized hospital service, e.g., obstetrics
   e. Shortage of midlevel providers and other health care professionals
   f. Professional isolation and lack of continuing education

3. State factors
   a. Lack of medical education opportunities in rural areas
   b. Underrepresentation of rural students in medical school(s)
   c. Tertiary care and subspecialty emphasis in medical education
   d. Absence of rural health office in state or local health departments

4. National factors
   a. Lack of federal programs, e.g., NHSC and CHC
   b. Lack of federal-state cooperative programs, e.g., AHEC
   c. Weak private and corporate support
   d. Federal immigration policies that restrict the flow of foreign medical graduates

local government in attempts to improve the delivery of rural primary care is also considered.

The final set of factors are those at the national level. Federal initiatives such as the NHSC and the CHC and MHC programs have experienced some successes, as have federal-state cooperative efforts, such as the AHEC program, and initiatives taken by various private foundations and corporations to provide health care services in rural areas. Federal immigration policies respecting FMGs also play a part in alleviating physician shortages in rural areas.

In the discussion that follows, we will illustrate the effects and interaction of the variables identified in tables 8.1 and 8.2, with examples drawn primarily from Arizona, the state with which we are most familiar, but also from selected other states. A few selected references to Canada will show similarities, even though the Canadian and U.S. health care systems differ markedly. Salient differences include policy options available to national and provincial governments, controls on hospital budgeting, and method

Table 8.2. Factors That Enhance Rural Physician Location:
Rural Pulls and Urban Pushes

1. Individual factors
   a. Rural origin of physicians or spouses
   b. Increasing number of female physicians
   c. Sufficient income to maintain a practice

2. Community factors
   a. Sufficient size and structure of service area populations
   b. Employment opportunities and viable economic climate
   c. Specialized cultural and educational opportunities
   d. Presence of a hospital within 30 minutes' travel time and of regional
      hospital programs and management contracts
   e. Availability of midlevel providers
   f. Opportunities for continuing education

3. State factors
   a. Opportunities for medical education in rural areas, e.g., AHEC training
      sites and rural residency programs
   b. Medical school recruitment of rural students
   c. Primary care emphasis in medical education
   d. State and local health departments including offices of rural health

4. National factors
   a. Federal programs, e.g., NHSC and CHC
   b. Federal-state cooperative programs, e.g., AHEC
   c. Private and corporate initiatives, e.g., United Mine Workers, Sears
      Roebuck Foundation, Kellogg Foundation, and Robert Wood Johnson
      Foundation
   d. Federal immigration policies that expand the flow of foreign medical graduates

of paying physicians. An important initial step is to define what is considered "rural." Rurality, as pointed out in chapter 2, is not a clearly defined concept. The extent to which an area is rural, the pattern of population distribution throughout a region, population characteristics, and many other factors affect the distribution of physicians and other health resources.

Arizona, the sixth largest in area of the fifty states, is divided into fifteen counties. Its population is largely urban—approximately 75 percent live in one of the two metropolitan counties, which include the Phoenix and Tucson metropolitan areas. Of the thirteen rural counties, four are classified as frontier areas, with population densities under six persons per square mile. There are three cities with populations between 25,000 and 50,000, and the rest of the state consists of small towns. Arizona has something of the configuration of a developing country, with a large capital city, a few provincial seats of government and commerce, and an extensive but thinly populated countryside. There is one medical school in the state, with all residency programs concentrated in either Tucson or Phoenix.

By contrast, North Carolina, a much smaller state geographically, is divided into 100 counties. Demographically it is a rural state, with 53 percent of its population in rural areas. Yet it has no frontier counties, nor does it have a city approaching the size of Phoenix (approximately 1 million people). With a population nearly twice that of Arizona (6 million to Arizona's 3.5 million), North Carolina has four medical schools and twenty-six distinct primary care residency programs distributed throughout the state. Of these, nine are in family practice (Mayer, 1988).

In addition to population distribution and density, other demographic elements, such as age structure, race/ethnicity, and income of the population, have significant implications for a health care system. For example, the presence of a larger number of the young and of older adults indicates that there will be high demand for health care services because they are both high-use groups. Racial and ethnic minorities are considered to be among high-risk populations, as are those in low-income groups.

Taking our case study of Arizona, its sizable elderly population is growing larger and also growing older. It is this increase in the elderly, many of whom live in rural areas, that will challenge the state's economy and its ability to provide needed services. The racial and ethnic composition of Arizona's people is diverse and requires culturally appropriate health services. In Indian population, Arizona ranks fourth in the United States, with a state proportion of 5.6 percent compared with 0.6 percent nationally. For people of Spanish heritage, the state ranks fourth, with a Hispanic population of 16.2 percent compared with 6.4 percent nationally. Only 2.8 percent of the state population is black, compared with 11.7 percent for the United States as a whole (Gordon, 1987, 7–9).

The state's economy ranked first in growth in personal income from 1975 to 1985, although a slowdown in the construction industry at the end of the decade changed this positive pattern. The economy of the thirteen nonmetropolitan counties has deteriorated over the years (Gordon, 1987, 9–10).

On a number of key measures of health care access, Arizonans are significantly worse off than most Americans. For example, 13 percent of Arizonans lack health insurance, compared to 9 percent nationally.

Twenty-five percent of Arizonans do not have a usual source of health care, compared to 18 percent nationally (Flinn Foundation, 1989). On access to prenatal care, the state ranks forty-fourth in the United States (Alan Guttmacher Institute, 1989).

Individual Factors

If the physician is to be "sovereign" in choosing where to provide services, then we must influence or change the attractiveness of markets. Otherwise, we must either change the physician's criteria of attractiveness or coerce the physician's choice (Feldstein, 1983). Many of the individual variables have to do with influencing the criteria of attractiveness of rural versus urban areas or recruiting into medicine those persons whose criteria are already likely to favor rural areas.

Place of origin. Physicians who come from rural areas, who graduate from rural high schools, or whose spouses are from rural areas are more likely to practice in rural areas than those who do not share these characteristics (Bible, 1970; Champion and Olsen, 1971; U.S. Department of Health and Human Services, 1980; Hassinger et al., 1979; Jonas, 1986; Leonardson et al., 1985; Long, 1975; Madison, 1980; Taylor et al., 1973; Tiedemann, 1987; Wilson, 1979). Women physicians are more likely than their male counterparts to choose rural practice locations (Burfield et al., 1986; Crowley et al., 1987; D'Elia and Johnson, 1980; Lorber, 1984). Given the increasing number and percentage of women in medicine in the United States, as well as in Canada (Adams, 1989), gender may prove to be an important factor in future physician location patterns.

Professional and social status. We can divide, somewhat crudely, the physician reward structure into three parts: prestige, economic benefits, and service. The mixture of these three is always complex, but in general in academic medical centers prestige predominates; in the secondary and tertiary centers outside academic medicine economic rewards hold sway; and in the primary care areas service is highlighted. Note that these three areas correspond, generally, to urban, suburban, and rural areas. Thus, the ideologies associated with practicing in different environments are important pushes or pulls influencing physician practice location. The causal direction is unclear. Rural physicians may embrace service and status/prestige at a community level as adequate rewards after practicing for several years (i.e., adjust their expectations). On the other hand, they may select rural locations because of the rewards they offer and the absence of pressures for other rewards, such as greater income or prestige in a national practice or research arena.

There is little documentation of the role played by status considerations in the choice of rural versus urban practice settings. Analysts suggest that status decreases the attractiveness of rural settings (Carter et al., 1974). Analysts also note that professional status varies by specialty, and the specialties associated with tertiary care are those carrying high status and high income.

Social status is associated with professional status, and both vary according to the geographic frame of reference, which may be local, regional, national, or international. Similarly, the sociological frame of reference would be "provincial" or "cosmopolitan." Small-town, rural physicians are likely to be accorded high professional and social status by others within the local frame of reference, yet implicitly have lower status than their urban professional colleagues. Thus, how status influences rural location depends on the perceived status needs of the individual physician. Does he or she like the idea of being a "pillar of the community," or does he or she yearn to be at the pinnacle of the profession? Rural residents confirm this distinction when they bypass local physicians in favor of urban counterparts for care that either could provide. Most of the forces acting to socialize students into the profession of medicine, to make them doctors, will pull physicians toward urban settings and away from rural settings (Carter et al., 1974; U.S. Department of Health and Human Services, 1980). One of the exceptions may be the type of doctor-patient relationship desired by the medical student and young physician (Hassinger et al., 1979). The ideal type for that relationship is a highly personalized, holistic one, deriving from the image of the family doctor, which is itself rooted in a traditional concept of community.

Income and lifestyle: Income, in most cases, discourages rural location. Rural physicians earn significantly less than their urban counterparts (Baker, 1988; McConnell and Tobias, 1986; Newhouse et al., 1982a; Schwartz et al., 1980; Wilson, 1979). It is not evident that a lower cost of living compensates for lower earnings.

If there is compensation, it is likely to be derived from the nebulous area of "lifestyle." Lifestyle or quality of life factors—such as educational opportunities, social and cultural amenities, environmental quality, and acceptable housing—clearly play a role in location choices (Coleman, 1976; U.S. Department of Health and Human Services, 1980; Hassinger et al., 1979). These lifestyle factors may be urban or rural pushes or pulls, depending on the individual physician and spouse. Similar findings on the importance of quality of life factors were recently reported by Canadian analysts (Anderson and Rosenberg, 1990).

Community Factors

Population size, distribution, and utilization patterns. Although individual physician characteristics are important in influencing whether physicians establish rural practices, so too are the characteristics of the rural communities themselves (Holmes and Miller, 1986). Having an adequate population or a population threshold of sufficient size to provide patients for a physician is a prerequisite. The adequacy of the population size is influenced by the population density, for even a numerically large population may not provide an attractive practice location if the residents are distributed over a large area (Berry and Garrison, 1958).

In a state such as Arizona, and in other states with large frontier areas, the fit between physician and rural community is often a poor one. There are few small to middle-sized cities that are able to compete with the suburbs of large metropolitan areas where young or established physicians are likely to settle. There are only three such cities in Arizona—Flagstaff, Sierra Vista, and Yuma—that are able to attract physicians, and a few resort-retirement towns also have succeeded in recruiting and retaining physicians.

Not only is the size of the population important, but so is understanding utilization patterns (Shannon et al., 1969; Weiss et al., 1971). For example, where a physician's patients come from and, conversely, which physicians are used by patients in a given geographic area or community are the factors that determine a physician's *market area.* Analyses using patient and hospital zip code data and other techniques measure hospital market areas (Garnick et al., 1987; Mayer, 1983). Similar analyses, including referral patterns, are needed for rural physicians and rural patients. This approach is important because the assumption that a physician cares for patients who live near his or her office may be misleading; for example, travel of rural residents to urban centers for care may be diagnosis-specific, or it may be influenced by the patient's social class. A common concern of rural hospital supporters is that the leaders in rural communities, although they want to retain their local hospital, often travel to urban centers for their own medical care.

Economic climate. The local population must also have the resources to support a physician. Even if a large rural population exists and needs medical care, a physician may hesitate to practice in a community if most of the population is unable to pay for medical services. Rural medical practices provide service, but the economic and business aspects of medical practice are an essential component of location decisions. Although the service orientation is often in the forefront when policy analysts consider the need for rural physicians, the market perspective may be a more important influence on a ⁻ ˙ιysician's location decision. This decision often entails an assess ˌnent of the future growth and development of the area.

Nonmetropolitan populations are economically disadvantaged relative to metropolitan populations, and the reasons appear to have more to do with underemployment than unemployment (Cordes, 1989). Even though there is a much higher incidence of poverty in rural or nonmetropolitan areas, there is less participation in income-supplement programs such as Aid to Families with Dependent Children (AFDC) and the Medicaid program. The proportion of the nonmetropolitan population that participates in AFDC is 3.7 percent compared to 4.9 percent for metropolitan population participation (Cordes, 1989). Medicaid program participation follows a similar pattern in that 25 percent of the rural poor qualify for Medicaid, compared to 43 percent of the urban poor (American Public Health Association, 1989). The large number of poor and uninsured persons in some rural areas discourages physicians from establishing and/or continuing practices.

Cultural and educational opportunities. The cultural, political, and religious conservatism for which small towns are stereotypically known may attract or inhibit physician location, depending on the orientation of the individual physician and spouse (Jonas, 1986).

In some states, including Arizona, there are special populations and special cultural opportunities that may attract physicians (Jonas, 1986; Langwell et al., 1985). The presence of American Indians and Hispanics in many rural areas of Arizona undoubtedly appeals to some physicians and their families. However, overall, small towns without exceptional recreational or cultural amenities, without great natural beauty, and without affluent retirees continue to struggle to recruit and retain physicians.

Practice characteristics in rural communities. Physicians in rural communities face a common set of problems. The smaller and more rural the town, the more likely it is that a physician will conduct a solo practice, with few if any colleagues nearby. This situation may result in a sense of professional, if not social, isolation. Although the absence of collegial discussion is a detriment, personal relationships with other community physicians may have either a positive or a negative influence, depending on individual compatibility.

There may also be fewer midlevel providers, such as nurse practitioners and physician assistants, available to support the physician. Secondary and tertiary care are likely to be frustratingly distant (Jonas, 1986; Leonardson et al., 1985; Mayer, 1988), as will be any medical school. Opportunities for continuing education will be severely limited. The physician may have no other physician with whom to share "call"—those times outside regular office hours, including nights and weekends, when the physician must respond to patient needs. When leaving town on business or for a vacation, the physician would have to attempt to find a "locum tenens," another physician who would replace her or him temporarily. Thus, the degree of rurality, with most of what it implies, can be seen as a push away for physician location (Cordes, 1989; Hewitt, 1989; Jonas, 1986; Leonardson et al., 1985; Northcott, 1980). The same factors account for the lack of appeal of rural areas in Canada (Anderson and Rosenberg, 1990).

Other community variables that tend to be a function of rurality include poverty (Langwell et al., 1985, 1987), and thus weak demand for health care; overall economic patterns (Cordes, 1989; Feldstein, 1983; Langwell et al., 1985); and the educational level and occupational distribution of the community (Cordes, 1989; Jonas, 1986). Research indicates that communities with a larger population, more physicians, a college, more white-collar employment, and a lower proportion of the population on farms are more likely to attract young physicians (Langwell et al., 1985). These can be considered factors that pull physicians to a rural community.

Of the variables examined at the community level, the increasing presence of hospital corporations in rural areas appears to hold promise for attracting physicians (Feldstein, 1983; Langwell et al., 1985). Large, urban-based hospitals have recently begun to expand their operations into rural areas (Tiedemann, 1987). The reasons for the entry of hospitals into rural health are clear—the large secondary and tertiary care centers need to expand their patient referral base, and they are doing so by entering into management contracts with rural community hospitals and clinics or by buying them outright; by establishing urgent care centers in small towns; or by establishing other kinds of referral links with local institutions.

In Arizona, large urban medical care organizations have rescued several rural hospitals that would otherwise have gone out of business. Some have been maintained as hospitals, while others have been converted into primary care clinics or urgent care centers. The immediate effects—namely, the infusion of capital and staff and the maintenance of previously threatened services— have fostered rural physician location. The urban organization provides an otherwise missing link between the potentially isolated rural physician and her or his urban counterparts, between the front line primary care provider and the specialty and tertiary care support that physicians have come to expect and to rely upon. In the short run, then, one would expect rural communities to welcome the urban organization and thereby to strengthen their ability to recruit and retain physicians.

The disadvantages of the presence of urban medical care organizations in rural settings lie more in the long run and are more difficult to assess. One can, nevertheless, begin to identify problems. For example, in one scenario a community health center is purchased by an outside corporation, and its local board of directors dissolves or becomes an advisory committee. An outside manager arrives, or the center's director becomes a corporate employee. Local control, local initiative, and community participation decrease or cease. In exchange, the community reaps economic and, perhaps, service benefits. But (as has already happened in a few cases in Arizona) should the clinic or hospital prove to have been a poor investment, it may be closed unless another buyer is found. The community may then be unprepared or unable to sustain the operation.

A case that illustrates the difficult trade-offs in establishing and maintaining medical care in an isolated rural community is the primary care center at Gila Bend in Arizona. Gila Bend is an agricultural town of 1,500, located on Interstate 8 midway between Phoenix and Yuma, approximately in the middle of a largely undeveloped expanse of open desert. The center was operated until 1989 by a Phoenix-based hospital. In addition to providing primary care services to the town, the center's emergency medical services (EMS) unit was responsible for almost 150 miles of the highway; so, in addition to the usual primary care provided, the center had to deal with a number of trauma cases from the highway as well as an array of agriculture-related injuries. The clinic was staffed by one physician assistant and an EMS team. A family practice resident from the Phoenix hospital spent one day a week at the center.

In 1989, the hospital decided to end its relationship with the Gila Bend clinic. It was then up to the town to sustain the operation and attempt to find a physician to practice there or, at least, to provide backup to the physician assistant. Although the townspeople mobilized themselves to try to save the clinic, it was problematic whether such a small town alone could sustain a physician. Yet Gila Bend is so far from any other health care services—120 miles from Yuma, 100 miles from Phoenix—that not to provide care places its population at considerable risk.

What occurred in Gila Bend, after the hospital withdrew from operation of the clinic in 1989, is an example of the difficulties as well as the creativity needed to continue to provide health care services to residents of a small community. Upon its withdrawal of responsibility, the hospital deeded the clinic and land to a community-based board of directors. Owing to the board's management inexperience, the clinic's primary care services became a responsibility of the town's municipal services, and clinic personnel became city employees. The clinic's EMS was taken over by a private ambulance company. During the two years of city management, the clinic operated at a financial loss. In the summer of 1991 responsibility was transferred back to the community-based board. The board, given its lack of clinic management experience, contracted with a federally funded CHC/CMC on the outskirts of metropolitan Phoenix not only to provide management services but also to recruit and supervise a physician assistant and to send its physician to Gila Bend for a semimonthly visit for consultation that would mitigate the isolation of the physician assistant. The town has continued to subsidize the clinic by keeping clinic personnel on the payroll. The exception is the midlevel provider, who is an employee of the contracted urban CHC/CMC (Hook, 1991).

Other linkages between urban and rural physicians, such as large multispecialty group practices, may play an increasingly important role in insuring the adequacy of the rural physician supply. These organizations can alter the context of analysis of rural physician supply by establishing a formal organizational framework to replace what has been predominantly an informal system of relationships. For example, a multispecialty group practice could place a physician in a rural community to insure that referrals come to their specialist. A physician placed in a rural community need not make a career commitment to the rural practice. A time limit may be part of the agreement, after which the physician is placed elsewhere in the organization. Such arrangements could provide explicit professional support and relationships, such as referral sources and coverage for the practice, thus meeting physicians' economic criteria for selecting rural locations. However, the rural poor and those in extremely low-density areas would continue to require special policy efforts and programs to address their needs. Short of some unforeseen changes in the nature of rural and/or urban life, the answers to physician maldistribution must be sought at levels beyond that of the community.

State Factors

Medical education. Several aspects of medical education are considered here at the state level because, as a matter of policy or practice, medical schools affect the practice of medicine regionally or throughout a state (Burfield et al., 1986) and are themselves affected by health policy and politics at the state level (Manard and Lewin, 1983). This is particularly true of public medical schools, which are typically mandated to meet certain expectations established through the legislative and political process (Hough and Marder, 1982; Kennedy et al., 1987; New York State Commission, 1986).

The medical school itself is almost always an urban institution. It is largely hospital-based, depending on sophisticated laboratories and technology, inpatient settings, and a highly specialized faculty. The student body, not surprisingly, is also highly urban.

In general, students from urban areas are overrepresented in medical schools (University of Arizona Admissions Committee, 1989). In 1988–1989, of 213 applicants to the University of Arizona College of Medicine, 201 were urban and 12, or 5.6 percent, were rural. The state population is about 25 percent rural. Of the entering class of 88, 5.7 percent were from rural areas, despite an admissions policy of overselecting for rural applicants. Rabinowitz (1983, 1988) and others (Dei Rossi, n.d.; Jonas, 1986; Mattson et al., 1973) have shown that admissions policies favoring rural applicants and applicants interested in family medicine will result in more physicians electing family medicine and rural practice locations. Without such policies, the urban origins of medical students reinforce tendencies to select urban practice locations.

The traditional curriculum offers little to interest students in underserved or rural areas or to encourage them seriously to consider practicing there. The excitement and satisfactions of medicine are more likely to be identified in the research laboratory, the intensive care unit, or the emergency room than in the outpatient clinic or local doctor's office. Nevertheless, curricular innovations and special programs, such as the AHEC program, have an impact on eventual specialty and practice location choices.

The AHEC program now operates in thirty-three states. Acting as the outreach arm of a medical school, this program establishes local centers that provide opportunities for medical students to spend time in the field with local physicians as teachers and role models, seeing patients in a primary care setting and learning about medical practice and community life in small towns.

In North Carolina, for example, the state has mandated its nine AHEC centers to provide all its family medicine residency training and much of its undergraduate education as well. The centers provide training in family and/or community medicine at eighty-four different sites throughout the state (Mayer, 1988). Arizona, with five AHEC centers and one medical school, offers training at twenty-five remote sites.

The Minnesota Rural Physician Associate Program provides a rural clerkship for nine of the twelve months of the third year to twenty-four student volunteers (Verby, 1988). Such a program would be difficult to establish at many medical schools, where the third year, which is the first clinical year of training, is typically firmly anchored in a tertiary care teaching hospital, preferably the school's own. At the University of New Mexico, a comparable program for first-year students provides six months of rural experience, along with a problem-based approach to the basic sciences as a substitute for the traditional first year, which is usually spent in basic sciences laboratories. Programs of this type move students out of the urban medical center and into rural communities (Baker, 1988; Blondell et al., 1989; Brearley et al., 1982; Glaser et al., 1982; Hale et al., 1979; Harris et al., 1982; Kaufman et al., 1983; Marder, 1974; Martin et al., 1971; Pust and Moher, 1983; Smith et al., 1982; West et al., 1982). There have also been attempts at the provincial level in Canada to make medical education more attuned to rural needs. In Ontario, for example, the Ministries of Health and Northern Affairs sponsor recruiting tours of medical schools and provide one- to three-month rural rotations for students, interns, and residents (Anderson and Rosenberg, 1990).

The medical school curriculum at the University of Arizona is not designed to give prominence to rural outreach programs. All third-year students are restricted to either Pima or Maricopa County (the state's two metropolitan statistical areas) for their clerkship rotations, with one exception: a community health center located sixty-five miles south of the medical school, on the Mexican border. The fourth year is elective. Students are encouraged to use these electives in their efforts to gain acceptance into residency programs. Thus rural rotations must compete with the attractions of residency program planning.

Shifts in emphasis of medical care from inpatient to ambulatory services will have an effect on medical education and will also shape individual choices of specialty and practice location in the future (Babbott et al., 1988). But at this moment, most students prefer a subspecialty to a primary care specialty, such as family practice, general pediatrics, or general internal medicine (Ciriacy et al., 1980; Cooper et al., 1972, 1975; Geyman et al., 1980; Gjerde and Parker, 1983; U.S. Department of Health and Human Services, 1980; Hecht and Farrell, 1982; Paiva et al., 1982). Students at osteopathic medical schools (D.O.s) are more likely to practice in rural areas than are graduates of allopathic medical schools (M.D.s)

(Baker, 1988; Bass and Paulman, 1983; Denslow et al., 1984; Jonas, 1986). A Canadian example from the province of Quebec indicates that physicians who work in salaried positions in publicly funded primary care community services are more likely to be female and to be located in rural areas than are physicians in private practice (Maheux et al., 1990).

The importance of monetary rewards for specialty choice and practice location choice is increased by the high cost of medical education (Holt, 1989; Mantovani et al., 1976; Parker and Sorensen, 1978; Yett and Sloan, 1974). The typical medical student graduates with a considerable debt burden, and this burden adds to the attractiveness of the high-compensation specialties, such as cardiology, radiology, and orthopedic surgery. Loan and scholarship programs counteract the effect of cost, but overall the need to finance education through subsequent earnings discourages rural location. The number of scholarships available through the NHSC, for example, has been greatly reduced.

Where a physician receives her or his graduate training strongly influences eventual practice location (Fein and Weber, 1971; U.S. Department of Health and Human Services, 1980; Held, 1973; Leonardson et al., 1985; Wunderman and Steiber, 1983; Yett and Sloan, 1974). Arizona retains 33 percent of its family practice residents. About half of these settle outside the Tucson and Phoenix metropolitan areas.

State and local health departments. Some states have expanded their roles in the direct provision of personal medical services in rural areas. Responsibilities of public health departments traditionally have been limited to communicable disease control, provision of maternal and child health services, environmental sanitation, health education, generation of vital statistics, and provision of laboratory services (Rosenblatt and Moscovice, 1982).

In North Carolina, for example, in the late 1970s, the role of health departments was expanded to include the provision of primary care services in rural areas. The State Health Services Division provided funds to twenty of the eighty-one local health departments to implement a variety of rural primary care programs (Miller et al., 1981; Tilson and Jellinek, 1981).

In Arizona, state law allows for several geopolitical forms of local health departments and local boards of health, a flexibility that accounts for variations in service delivery mechanisms.

Because Arizona's fifteen counties vary greatly in size, population, and resources, the county health departments differ in scope of services provided (Arizona Statewide Health Coordinating Council, 1985). Unlike the two urban counties, the thirteen rural counties have very limited direct primary care services provided by county health departments.

The proportion of primary care physicians in private practice in Arizona's rural counties has decreased considerably over the years, from 21.7 percent of the state total in 1960 to 13.9 percent in 1984. From 1960 to 1984, rural counties as a whole experienced an 8 percent deterioration in the ratio of physicians to population, while the two urban counties experienced a 24.4 percent increase (Arizona Statewide Health Coordinating Council, 1985, 8–4). Compounding this situation is the decreasing number of physicians available in rural counties to deliver babies, owing largely to the high cost of malpractice insurance and threat of suit (Gordon et al., 1987; Gordon and Higgins, 1991). A rural physicians' subsidy to offset the cost of malpractice premiums was allocated by the 1989 Arizona Legislature. The intent of the assistance bill was to provide immediate help in an attempt to keep rural physicians from curtailing their obstetric practice. The diminishing supply of rural physicians available to do deliveries may push state and local health departments to work cooperatively and begin to play a more central role in providing health services in rural areas.

National Factors

The decision-making framework discussed at the individual, community, and state levels can be extended to include systematic efforts that influence physician decision-making, such as the explicit policies and programs of the federal government. The various national efforts to influence physician supply and distribution can be divided into two basic strategies. The first is a regulatory approach characterized by central planning, mandated programs, and direct measurement of geographically underserved areas as a basis for targeting areas most in need. This approach has tended to be more micro-oriented and direct, focusing on individual physicians or on the areas in which these physicians were needed. The second strategy relies more on market mechanisms and the incremental effects of numerous decisions over time to bring about a diffusion of physicians to rural areas. In theory, the increasing supply of physicians will increase competition among physicians in the most desirable communities and result in more physicians establishing practices in less competitive areas, such as many rural communities. This approach is more macro-oriented and indirect, depending on the consequences of an increasing physician supply throughout the whole system. The results of the macroapproach have been mixed (Fruen and Cantwell, 1982; Hynes and Givner, 1983; Newhouse et al., 1982b; Schwartz et al., 1980, 1988; Williams et al., 1983). Both these strategies aim to bring about the same results: a more equitable distribution of physicians in rural areas.

Federal programs. Under the regulatory strategy, the federal government has launched two major funding initiatives to help improve health care delivery in rural areas. The first is in the training of primary care providers; the second is in developing and expanding primary care service delivery programs (Lee et al., 1976).

The training of primary care providers was assisted by the Health Professions Educational Assistance Act of 1976 (P. L. 94-484), which required medical schools wishing to be recipients of federal capitation grants to fill at least 50 percent of first-year residency training slots in the primary care specialties. In this act, primary care specialties were recognized as general internal medicine, pediatrics, and family medicine. As a consequence, family medicine residencies were considerably expanded.

There was also emphasis on creating training programs for new kinds of primary care practitioners, most notably physician assistants and nurse practitioners, often called midlevel practitioners (Schneller, 1976). On the whole, midlevels have been more responsive than physicians in serving in rural areas. For example, in 1987 the ratio of physician assistants in Arizona's rural counties was 8 per 100,000, compared to 6 per 100,000 in the urban counties (Gordon, 1987).

Programs that the federal government initiated in the 1970s were intended to assure access to health care for rural residents. They included the CHC, AHEC, and NHSC programs. These rural initiatives often met pressing short-term needs, such as temporarily placing physicians in areas lacking health personnel. The two federal programs that provided the majority of the funding and workforce for rural areas were the NHSC and CHC initiatives (Rosenblatt and Moscovice, 1982).

The NHSC was created in 1971 and differed from previous federal efforts because it took direct action in placing health providers in shortage areas rather than funding development of health care delivery programs. In 1976, support for the NHSC was expanded to include a large scholarship program, which would insure a steady flow of recent medical graduates for work in federally sponsored primary care programs. Recipients of NHSC scholarships were required to practice in a designated underserved area for one year of obligated service as payment for each year of scholarship assistance, with a minimum of two years.

The Omnibus Budget Reconciliation Act of 1981 (P.L. 97-35) considerably reduced funding for the NHSC. This policy decision resulted from the general shift from an expansive and regulatory federal role in health care in the 1970s to a market-driven, competitive approach in the 1980s. The shift was enhanced by studies noting a growing physician surplus (U.S. Department of Health and Human Services, 1980), which ironically was reported just six years after the federal government had announced a national physician shortage (Hafferty, 1986).

The withering of the NHSC is contrary to positive evaluations of the program (Rosenblatt and Moscovice, 1978, 1979, 1980; U.S. Department of Health and Human Services, 1984; U.S. Department of Health and Human Services, 1986a,b), which clearly indicate that placement of physicians and other health care personnel in rural communities increased the availability of primary health care services. Research showed that the NHSC improved the distribution of health resources between rural and urban areas, and among rural areas (Cromley, 1989; Horner, 1988).

Langwell and her colleagues (1986a,b) concluded that physicians with NHSC experience, when compared to physicians without this experience, were more likely to choose to locate their practices in communities that were in greater need of health care services. According to advocates of the regulatory approach, and based on its past positive record of placing providers in underserved rural areas, the NHSC needs to be redefined, revitalized, and strengthened.

The CHC program, which grew out of a 1964 Office of Economic Opportunity–initiated project called Neighborhood Health Centers, is another important federal program. Centers were designed to provide access to ambulatory care in rural and inner-city areas. Those primary care centers that qualify as CHCs or MHCs receive federal grants under Section 329 and/or Section 330 of Title III of the U.S. Public Health Service Act (as amended). In recent years, the CHC program has increasingly focused on rural areas. CHCs serve predominantly low-income people, who suffer numerous barriers to care. The available evidence indicates that the policy has had a positive effect on the health status of rural populations. There is also partial evidence that the policy has been cost-effective (Davis et al., 1981; Horner, 1988).

Federal-state initiative. The AHEC program is a federal-state cooperative effort that has had a positive effect on physician distribution. The aim of the program is to decentralize health professional educational training opportunities, link rural health providers and facilities with large urban health resource centers, and work with the NHSC to place physicians in underserved areas (Sheps and Bachar, 1981). After an AHEC is established, it is expected to seek and receive funding from state and other nonfederal funding sources. Many states have been successful in receiving this funding.

AHECs provide an opportunity for students to gain firsthand experience in medicine, health care, and community life in a rural underserved area. This approach has been successful according to studies that show that health professionals are more likely to choose to practice in an area where they have received training (McEniry et al.,1988).

Private and corporate initiatives. Private-sector initiatives also play a role in bringing physicians to rural areas. One of the early nongovernmental attempts at providing health services in rural areas was undertaken by the United Mine Workers of America. Their welfare and retirement fund supported the Miner's Medical Program, which operated in the Appalachian region from 1946 to 1978 (E. W. Boyd et al., 1982). Other private efforts include the Sears Roebuck Foundation, the W. K. Kellogg Foundation, and the Robert Wood Johnson Foundation (DeFriese and Ricketts, 1989; Kane et al., 1975; Moscovice and Rosenblatt, 1982a).

From 1957 to 1970, the Sears Roebuck Foundation developed and equipped clinics in 163 rural communities to help improve the recruitment and retention of physicians. Evaluation of the program indicated 20 percent of the 163 rural areas that had facilities were still not able to attract physicians to their communities, and retention among recruited physicians was a continuing problem (Kane et al., 1975). The program's lack of success pointed out that facilities alone were not a sufficient solution to bringing health care to rural areas.

The W. K. Kellogg Foundation undertook a variety of primary care initiatives in rural communities called Innovations in Ambulatory Primary Care. The program included grants to twenty-three organizations for the development of innovative programs for the delivery of primary care services to rural populations. A summary of eight case studies was published (Bisbee, 1982), although no standardized evaluation was undertaken (DeFriese and Ricketts, 1989).

The Robert Wood Johnson Foundation funded an initiative, 1975–1979, to develop multidisciplinary team practices that would produce stable primary care centers throughout rural America. The Rural Practice Project provided grants to thirteen separate clinic programs, each of which included a physician and health administrator team. The goal for each team was to provide the core of a successful, community-responsive, self-sufficient rural practice. Even though it was expensive to maintain a full-time administrator at each site, all of the practices have survived (DeFriese and Ricketts, 1989; Moscovice and Rosenblatt, 1982b).

Federal immigration policies. FMGs have an effect on physician supply and distribution in rural areas. Although the migration of alien physicians to the United States is not a new phenomenon, the flow of immigrants was relatively small until the late 1960s. Analysts subsequently reported estimates of as many as 40,000 physicians a year who took part in international migrations, with the United States being a major attraction center (Gish, 1971).

The number of FMGs in the U.S. physician supply increased dramatically over the 1970–1979 period. They comprised 13 percent of all physicians in the United States in 1963 and almost 22 percent of all physicians in 1974 (American Medical Association, 1975). Moreover, 33 percent of all U.S. residencies were filled by FMGs in 1970 (American Medical Association, 1971). The heavy influx of FMGs in the 1960s and 1970s would not have occurred without a demand for their services. In the post-World War II era the demand for health care in the United States increased, initially because of the rapid spread of private health insurance coverage and later because of the enactment of Medicare and Medicaid legislation in 1965 (Carnegie Council, 1976), which provided public funds for services to the aged and the poor.

Immigration laws were modified in 1965 and 1970 to help facilitate the flow of FMGs into the United States to meet the increased demand. By 1976, an increase in the supply of U.S. medical graduates had prompted tightening of visa regulations in an attempt to make it more difficult for FMGs to enter the United States or to remain here. More recent legislation and tightened examination procedures have further restricted the supply. Consequently, the percentage of FMGs in U.S. residency training programs has been declining steadily since 1980, when it was at 19.8 percent. By 1987, the percentage of FMG residents had decreased to 15.6 percent (Crowley et al., 1987). By 1988, the figure was close to 13 percent (Sandrick, 1988). Some analysts predict few FMGs will be able to compete with U.S. medical graduates for residency slots in the future (Mick and Worobey, 1986). Unless there are changes in the restrictive policies, it is unlikely that this declining trend will be reversed.

FMGs tend to work in areas less desirable to American physicians, such as central city hospitals and rural areas. They are found in greater relative proportions in rural America and accounted for nearly 40 percent of the overall physician expansion in nonmetropolitan areas from 1970 to 1979 (U.S. Department of Health and Human Services, Bureau of Health Professions, 1983). Female FMGs locate in greater relative numbers in rural areas than their male FMG or female U.S. medical graduate counterparts (D'Elia and Johnson, 1980). FMGs generally are more evenly distributed relative to the population they serve (Politzer et al., 1978). The supply of FMGs increased in all types of small rural counties over the period 1975 to 1985 (Kindig and Movassaghi, 1989; Swearinger and Perrin, 1977). However, even with this expansion in physician availability in small rural counties, these areas were still relatively underserved (Kindig and Movassaghi, 1989).

This workforce, who generally were willing to work for less money and to practice in areas from which American-trained physicians shy away (Sandrick, 1988; Swearinger and Perrin, 1977), has made a considerable contribution to the medical care of the American public, both in poor urban areas and in rural areas that have experienced a shortage of physicians (Butter et al., 1978; Koska, 1988; Studnicki et al., 1976). FMGs serve, in effect, as a reserve physician supply in the American health system and provide services to potentially deprived populations. Evidence from Canada suggests a similar pattern. In some provinces, FMGs constitute up to 60 percent of the rural practitioners (Adams, 1989). Changes in FMG immigration policy, and other policies that attempt to curtail the increase of future FMG participation in the U.S. health delivery system, could have a negative impact on the underserved urban and rural areas where FMGs fill the gap.

Summary

In this chapter a myriad of factors that influence physician distribution were summarized as rural or urban pushes or pulls. The framework is intended to encourage understanding of the complex forces that operate at several levels. In many cases, but not always, the factors that push physicians away from urban areas and those that pull physicians to rural areas are the same. The framework suggests that changes at one level can affect the whole. This complicates policy efforts directed at increasing rural location of physicians. Such policies must account for the complex interplay among rural and urban pushes and pulls that is generated at the individual, community, state, and national levels. Perhaps most important is the apparent failure to build on the successes of programs that have been effective at establishing physicians in underserved rural locations.

Chapter 9

Rural Primary Care Programs in the United States
A Decade of Change

THOMAS C. RICKETTS AND

ELIZABETH CROMARTIE

The push to make health care readily available to a significant portion of the American public was, and is, important to the ten million rural residents without a regular source of care, to the sixteen million who live in communities without adequate primary care providers, and to the almost seventeen million who suffer from some form of chronic or serious illness (Norton and McManus, 1989). This public policy has been typically American in that it has combined several political and social viewpoints into a single structural solution. The single solution of placing health centers and health personnel in underserved areas has produced its own plural system of organizational forms. The comparison and contrast of those forms was the topic of the National Evaluation of Rural Primary Care Programs that the University of North Carolina Health Services Research Center conducted during the period 1977–1985 with support from the Robert Wood Johnson Foundation and the U.S. Department of Health and Human Services. In-depth descriptions of the National Evaluation have appeared as reports, journal articles, and dissertations.[1] The project described in this chapter represents an extension of that evaluation by analyzing one of the four samples selected by the National

---

[1] Staff from the National Evaluation produced 15 journal articles and data were used in five dissertations and several journal articles published by independent researchers using public use data files fromthe National Evaluation. Individual citations in this chapter will focus on prominent publications from the Evaluation.

Evaluation to determine patterns of development and change in subsidized or once-subsidized rural centers.

The pressure on distributive social policies to produce their intended effects as efficiently as possible was an implicit reason for the inception of the National Evaluation. This economic and political reality remains part of the policy environment of the programs. However, neither the National Evaluation nor this analysis is intended to focus on efficiency. The intention of this analysis is to develop new understanding of the long-term natural history of programs that were born in subsidy, and have had to survive either by continuing to generate that subsidy or by weaning themselves away from external subvention to become freestanding programs. Not all have survived as they intended, as we shall see.

The National Evaluation of Rural
Primary Care Programs

The National Evaluation of Rural Primary Care Programs was undertaken in 1977 by the Health Services Research Center of the University of North Carolina at Chapel Hill. The goal of the project was to determine the overall effect of the wide array of programs that were meant to improve access to primary care among rural, underserved populations. The National Evaluation began with an effort to establish a comprehensive inventory of subsidized rural primary care programs sponsored by both public and private sources in the United States. At the outset of the study, listings of projects that were supported by private foundations, state governmental agencies, and federal programs were compiled. The resulting inventory of programs included the names of over 1,300 separate organizations or programs supposedly offering primary health care services and having received some form of subsidy in order to begin or continue their operations. Efforts to estimate the extent to which the inventory actually included all of the programs that were of interest were made in several states, where experts known to have firsthand local knowledge of such programs were asked to examine the inventory compiled by the project for their state. Comprehensive information was obtained from officials in California, West Virginia, North Carolina, New Mexico, Washington, and Florida, and those listings were compared to the evaluation's listings. From this process it was estimated that the national inventory contained more than 90 percent of all of the potential rural primary care programs that had had some form of subsidization at some time in their operation. Using the inventory, a national mail survey was conducted of all known potential rural primary care programs that had been subsidized at some time in their history; 998 could be located and telephoned. The survey process led to the identification of 627 programs that delivered primary care at least four days per week in a rural community and either were receiving external support or had received it at some time in their history.

A central objective of the project was the confirmation of the existence of a typology of rural primary care clinics. Sheps and his colleagues (Sheps and Bachar, 1981) had suggested that the overwhelming majority of subsidized rural primary care programs fell into five classifications: comprehensive health centers, organized group practices, institutional extensions, primary care centers, and traditional solo or partnership practices. The project wished to determine the degree to which these programs met the intentions of their original funders in terms of organizational viability, access to services, and access to care for the population in the communities.

Collecting data to measure impacts on access by the programs required extensive and costly community surveys. The project chose to focus its in-depth studies in regions of the country where levels of underservice were highest. Because funds restricted the number of site visits that were possible, the project chose to conduct the community surveys and in-depth studies of the program through site visits to a sample of forty programs that were chosen to represent the three most common organizational forms identified in the evaluation. This roughly approximated the southeastern and western parts of the United States. The exclusion of the northeastern and northwestern portions of the nation was intended to focus the study on those regions of the country where problems of access to services for minorities and underserved populations had been determined to be greatest. The selection of the forty sites was made as part of the selection of a nationally representative sample of 193 programs. The map in fig. 9.1 locates the forty sites that were chosen for in-depth site visits as well as eight comparison communities that were matched to the program sites in size and degree of health personnel need. The comparison sites had been in the process of planning for or seeking support for a subsidized clinic during 1979.

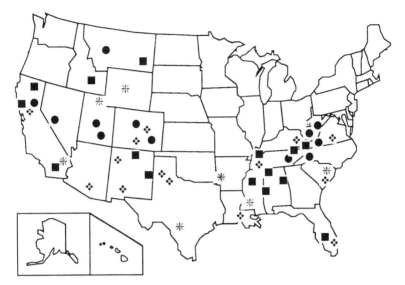

Fig. 9.1. Location of study sites for National Evaluation of Rural Primary Care Programs.
Key: ❖ = community health center, ● = organized group practice, ■ = primary care center, ✳ = comparison community.
Source: North Carolina Rural Health Research Program, Health Services Research Center, University of North Carolina at Chapel Hill.

The forty programs in the group were visited in 1980 and 1981 by teams from the Health Services Research Center with participation by project staff of the Robert Wood Johnson Foundation and the Office of the Assistant Secretary for Health. Thirty-six of the forty programs were also the target of community surveys of users and nonusers of the target clinics. These surveys, of approximately 250 adults and 125 children in each community, were meant to develop indexes of access for users compared to nonusers. The surveys were also completed in the eight comparison communities.

Findings from the Original Study

The study confirmed the central hypothesis of the evaluation, that there would be a limited number of organizational forms in the universe of organizations that delivered primary care in rural communities. The data supported the division of the forms into three major types, with a small number of programs that could be called "institutional extensions," usually of hospitals and large multispecialty clinics, and a small residual group of unclassifiable forms; these two groups accounted for less than 10 percent of the total universe of programs. The three principal forms and their characteristics included:

1. *Comprehensive health centers (CHCs):* Primary health care programs characterized by comprehensive program development on a relatively large scale, together with substantial community involvement and control. Social and health objectives were to be achieved by a relatively broad range of nonclinical services to support and extend the impact of basic medical services. Examples included the neighborhood health centers and family health centers (mainly supported by the Department of Health and Human Services), of which a sizable number served rural populations.
2. *Organized group practices (OGPs):* Primary health care programs that consist of at least two full-time physicians in group practice operating autonomously, through a pooled income arrangement, not providing any outreach services. Some, like the practices fostered and supported by the Robert Wood Johnson Foundation Rural Practice Project, emphasized leadership by physicians, sophisticated administration, and staff development.
3. *Primary care centers (PCCs):* Smaller primary health care programs stimulated and/or subsidized by indigenous community initiative, with or without financial assistance from outside the community, and often involving the use of new health professionals with physician backup, on site or elsewhere. There was usually no formal institutional affiliation.

The analysis of these three organizational types and their performance led to the following eight observations and conclusions:

1. The classification of programs by organizational form followed an explicit algorithm and incorporated most of the principal criteria for program selection by public or private funding agencies. Hence, the differences among these organizational forms were usually *by design* and occurred in response to the

mandatory requirements of a funding agency. Moreover, certain organizational forms of practice tended to be associated with particular types of communities, to offer a distinctive set of services, and to have a particular set of financial policies regarding patient payment for services received (Sheps et al., 1983).

2. Organizational forms differ in financial performance after controlling for community characteristics. CHCs have higher costs and lower efficiency; OGPs have lower costs and greater efficiency; PCCs are intermediate between the other two types with respect to both of these variables (Bradham et al., 1985).

3. When faced with reductions in subsidy, rural primary care programs attempt to increase revenues before cutting costs and reducing services (University of North Carolina Health Services Research Center, 1985).

4. The competitive environments of subsidized rural PCCs can be classified into two categories: isolated and underserved. The centers have a variety of options available to them as they consider competitive reactions to alternative primary care resources in their communities. These revolve around managerial actions to reduce costs or to increase revenues or a combination of both. The choices made by the centers tend to relate to either (a) their perceived clinical mission (as a comprehensive program targeted to specific subpopulations), (b) their practice organization (emphasizing structural access to care), or (c) their providers' patterns of practice (emphasizing hospital practice or screening, prevention, and diagnosis versus conventional episodic care) (University of North Carolina Health Services Research Center, 1985).

5. There are significant differences between physicians and nurse practitioners or physician assistants in the way each views and reacts to service in rural primary care practice situations. New health practitioners are more likely to view such settings as a suitable place to fulfill their long-term career aspirations, and are more likely to, in fact, stay. Physicians generally view service in rural, subsidized health care programs as a temporary, less than optimal professional employment situation. Physicians' intentions to leave can be influenced by the organizational structures of these primary care centers. The data indicate that, where physi-

cians have the ability to modify the structure and operation of the centers, physicians in these centers report higher levels of work satisfaction and higher levels of retention after any obligated service commitments are met (University of North Carolina Health Services Research Center, 1983).

6. The type and source of subsidy greatly affect the structure, operation, and fiscal stability of programs. The extent of subsidy in the centers is related to the costs of care. For every $100,000 in program subsidy, the average increase in costs (per encounter) of care is $0.70. The extent to which the state Medicaid program covers the poor has a strong effect on the ability of the programs to cover costs as does the degree to which programs apply sliding fee schedules.

7. Access to care in subsidized rural PCCs, measured in terms of use of services in relation to symptoms and disability rates, was higher for users of the sponsored clinics than for nonusers in the surveyed communities. However, statistical significance for the comparisons was reached only for children on a measure of use related to disability and time spent in the hospital.

8. Satisfaction with care was higher in all communities with subsidized programs when compared to similar communities without such programs, and there were higher levels of satisfaction among program users than among nonusers where the programs offered a broader array of clinical and support services.

One of the principal criteria for inclusion in the study was the fact that the programs were receiving subsidies at the time of the survey or had received them in the recent past. Over half of the programs were started in 1975 or later and three-quarters after 1971. One hundred and fifty seven (81.3 percent) were receiving some form of federal funding or personnel support at the time of the survey in 1981; 16 (8.3 percent) were receiving some form of private foundation funding; 44 (22.8 percent) were receiving some form of nonfederal governmental funding; and 19 (9.8 percent) were receiving some private or local funding. The funding sources for the programs did not vary significantly among regions of the country. Programs in the west were slightly more likely to receive migrant health, local, and Comprehensive Educational and Training Act (CETA) subsidies, whereas those in the southeast were slightly more likely to receive funding from the Community Health Centers Program, CETA, or "other" federal programs. The pattern of subsidy among organizational forms showed CHCs far more likely to receive Migrant Health Center (MHC) (Section 329) and CHC (Section 330) support, whereas PCCs were subsidized much more often from state and local governments and local civic organizations. Programs also reported receiving funding from now-defunct programs, including the Rural Health Initiative (RHI) and Health Underserved Rural Areas (HURA) projects, which were folded into the CHC funding program during the late 1970s.

A number of combinations of subsidy occurred more frequently than others. They included

1. National Health Service Corps   111 programs (57.5 percent)
   (NHS) alone or with "other"
   federal subsidy
2. "Other" federal subsidy alone   21 programs (10.9 percent)
3. NHSC with RHI/HURA   14 programs (7.3 percent)
4. RHI/HURA alone   12 programs (6.2 percent)

Initial Follow-up Surveys

Because of the rapid pace of change in the political environment of direct-service delivery programs supported by the federal government that occurred when the Reagan Administration came into office, it was decided to survey the 193 programs in the Tier II sample again during the summer of 1982. Contact was made with 184 (95 percent) of the programs. Nine of the 193 had closed during the year and a half period between surveys. Four of the 184 still operating chose not to respond to the 1982 survey. The results of this follow-up were reported in the *American Journal of Public Health* (Ricketts et al., 1984). The programs did face subsidy reductions during the period 1980–1982, but the cuts were not applied across the board as had been expected. Selected programs had their funding canceled or were forced to merge with other programs. One hundred and four of the responding programs suffered funding cuts, but forty-three had their funding levels raised. Where there were cuts, the programs generally chose to reduce costs rather than raise charges. A significant number of programs

(n = 41) did add income-generating services, including X-ray, laboratory, and pharmacy services. Cost reduction was achieved through staff reduction, cutbacks in ancillary services, or internal budget shifting rather than a reduction in primary care service content, although there was a net reduction in the number of programs offering evening and weekend hours, transportation, and twenty-four-hour telephone coverage. The overall result of changes in the programs' environments produced general belt-tightening, but the clinics proved to be resilient enough to absorb the relatively small shocks of the first years of the Reagan presidency.

First Provider Follow-up

In the original study of providers, 426 physicians in the 192 programs employing M.D.s or D.O.s, and 182 nurse practitioners or physician assistants responded to mail and telephone surveys. Those surveys gathered data describing the providers' backgrounds, training, and content of practice in the programs. A section of the survey elicited opinions concerning the practitioners' degree of satisfaction with the programs, the communities, and their practice. Finally, physicians were asked their intentions to practice in rural areas when they began training, began practice in the study site, and in the near future. These data were summarized in a series of variables that described recruitment and retention scores for each program and tenure for each provider; a series of independent variables that described the provider's background and whether he or she was in the NHSC or obligated for rural service through another program; and the environments, the organization, and the level of satisfaction with components of the practice and environment.

The original study had found that new health practitioners and physicians were equal in terms of their level of satisfaction with rural practice but that the nonphysicians intended to stay longer in rural areas. The correlates of satisfaction among physicians were their degree of involvement in local community activities and whether they had made a long-term housing commitment in the community. The analysis of the dependent variables produced mixed results. The individual characteristics associated with physicians' current career commitments were found to be being male, being married, and the absence of having had certain practice-relevant experiences—such as previous training in a rural area, membership in the NHSC, or a service-obligated practice. Expectations of retention for physicians were also associated with working in a program with more limited hours of available service and a professional practice environment characterized by a supply of health resources that was complementary to the practice of primary care. The community environment characteristic promoting retention was a relatively low proportion of Hispanics in the population, low proportions of persons below the poverty level, but rather higher proportions of nonwhites. The most marked individual correlate of initial career longevity expectations was NHSC status. Other individual factors were a housing investment index, a community commitment index, and the workload, expressed in terms of patients seen per week. Because NHSC status is associated with intention to stay at the beginning of rural practice, but not the intention to leave after a fixed period as expressed at the beginning of practice, it is suggested that physicians who are not in the corps are likely to choose rural practices with the intention of staying there, whereas corps physicians are either initially disposed to leave or undecided.

In 1985 the smaller sample of site-visited programs were recontacted to determine the location and practice status of the originally surveyed physicians. Included in the data set had been 126 physicians; 105 were located in 1985. At the time of recontact only nine of the physicians (five were D.O.s) were not in primary care and all nine had moved out of their 1980 communities. The overall retention in the program communities was 53%, with 48% of NHSC-obligated physicians remaining and 57% of non-corps M.D.s or D.O.s staying. The analysis of the retention patterns found little relationship between type of medical school or residency training and retention in the communities, nor were there significant differences in the patterns of correlation with the individual characteristics of the physicians or the environmental or organizational variables.

A more detailed analysis of the provider data with a focus on the role of the NHSC in provider retention in rural primary care centers was performed in 1989 by Donald Pathman, M.D., an associate of the Rural Health Research Program. That analysis found that, after controlling for the younger ages of NHSC physicians and the more sparsely populated locations of NHSC practices, rural corps physicians are found to be no different in their initial retention plan than non-NHSC physicians. This contradicts the notion that NHSC physicians are initially less committed to rural practice because they are obligated for service. Also, after controlling for differential initial retention plans, NHSC physicians are still more likely to leave rural practice after their obligations are completed than are non-corps physicians. The theory that NHSC experience adversely affects physician retention was, therefore, supported. The data support the policy options of recruiting older physicians and physicians with rural backgrounds to improve retention in rural communities and to examine and remedy problems in the structure and organization of the corps.

1989–1990 Follow-up Study Design

Because of the extensive longitudinal data that had been collected and maintained on the forty programs in the original evaluation, it was determined that a follow-up survey would allow us to gather a picture of the changes that had occurred in rural primary care programs since the early 1980s. A survey instrument was developed for a telephone survey of the programs and sites to be administered in mid-1989. Within the scheduled deadline for a coordinated survey, program contacts were identified for over half of the study sample of forty programs and all of the comparison sites; however, for slightly less than half of the programs effective contact was made difficult by changes that had occurred in the programs. The administration of the survey was delayed until the project staff were confident that they had willing informants in at least thirty-six of the programs. Interviews were conducted via telephone and mail survey forms were sent to all of the programs. By May 1990, thirty programs had completed the full mailed questionnaire. For those ten programs that did not respond via mail or refused a full telephone survey, additional telephone calls were made to other informants at the programs to elicit a minimum data set to allow for basic description of the program and its progress. Five of the programs responded to a full telephone survey and provided complete or nearly complete data; five programs responded to a limited number of questions or provided partial data. Informants who had worked with the two closed programs were located and interviewed (program administrator for duration of project for program #10786, and community leader and local hospital administrator for program #10202). Through this method, all forty programs have contributed a minimum data set to the research team.

Changes in the Environments
of the Programs

Rural clinics and rural primary care programs developed rapidly during the late 1960s and 1970s owing mostly to the availability of federal funds for Neighborhood, then Community Health Centers. From 1971, the NHSC was expanding its field strength until it reached a peak of 3,304 practitioners in 1986; programs in family medicine were opening, and the output of new family physicians grew to approximately 1,200 per year before steadying at that level in 1985. The corps met with strong resistance in Reagan-era budgets and present appropriations anticipate a phasing-down of the program. New scholarship awards have been reduced to 49 in 1989, down from a peak of 6,408 in 1979, and 937 in 1983, the last year that the program received significant funding for new students. The reduction in support for the program is largely a result of the interpretation of personnel distribution studies that predicted a physician surplus and extrapolated those results into rural areas (Schwartz et al., 1980; Newhouse, 1982; Newhouse et al., 1982a,b). In truth, physicians have not moved into nonmetropolitan areas, especially the smallest (Kindig and Movassaghi, 1989), and nonmetropolitan America has not seen the rate of overall growth in physician supply that metropolitan and suburban America has experienced.

The total number of subsidized rural primary care programs increased to approximately 1,500 different entities administering one or more delivery sites during the period 1980 to 1982, partly as a result of the continuing flow of federal support (National Rural Health Association, 1988b). In 1982, there was a distinct change in federal policy toward support for social programs. Initially, the CHC program was to be included in a primary care block grant that was to be funded at 75 percent of the total 1981 level of funding for all categorical programs included under the block grant. Only one state, West Virginia, opted to accept the block grant arrangement, and the remaining states more or less actively supported the independence of the CHCs and MHCs through their congressmen or state health agencies. Despite repeated efforts by the Reagan Administration to cancel funding for the Section 329 (MHC) and Section 330 (CHC) programs, they remained funded at maintenance levels throughout the 1980s, holding at $325 million in 1980 through 1985 and currently at $463 million in the FY 1990 budget. However, adjusted for inflation and subtracting the special projects provisions from the current appropriation, real funding for CHCs has dropped. The number of CHCs funded in 1988, 526, has dropped from 608 in 1984. Most of the closures or mergers have been in rural centers, the number of which dropped from 399 in 1984 to 319 in 1988, a 20 percent decrease.

CHC funding is a principal source, but only one of several sources, of support for rural primary care programs. There is, however, no survey of current and recent changes in state and private funding programs for such programs. Major philanthropies have continued to support programs and projects in existing sites. For example, the Robert Wood Johnson Foundation and the W. K. Kellogg Foundation remain very active in support of the projects. Several states remain active in supporting clinics and programs, either directly or indirectly. (See chapter 8 for discussions of nonfederal initiatives.) These initiatives, however, do not approach the level of support and encouragement of program development and operation during the 1970s.

The Area Health Education Centers (AHEC) program has survived since its inception in 1972 as one way to develop state- and regional-level linkages between academic health centers and practicing physicians in rural areas. The impact of AHECs on rural physician location decisions has been hard to assess and their use of primary care centers and programs is very unevenly recorded (American Institutes for Research, 1990). Several new AHECs were funded during the period between studies but their impacts are not well understood.

Medicaid and Medicare provide very significant amounts of revenue for the rural primary care centers, as almost 45 percent of total patient revenue for the programs came from these sources in 1980 (see chapter 11 for more on the financial aspects of rural health.) However, Medicaid payment levels are traditionally lower than average costs and the Medicare program pays rural physicians lower rates than urban physicians. The size of the rural-urban payment differential in Medicare for physician services has increased over the past decade. One planned mechanism to support primary care services in rural areas through the Medicaid and Medicare programs was included in the Rural Health Clinics Act (P.L. 95-210), which allowed for direct reimbursement of nurse practitioners, certified nurse midwives, and physician assistants. Clinics could be certified for this reimbursement if they were located in underserved areas and were primarily primary care providers. There were 470 certified rural health centers in April 1989, with 60 percent of these concentrated in ten states (California, Georgia, Maine, New Mexico, New York, North Carolina, Pennsylvania, South Dakota, Tennessee, West Virginia). This number is far lower than had been expected when the program was begun; poor administrative coordination between agencies and little incentive for the programs to apply for designation have been cited as reasons for the low participation. The regulations for designation have recently been liberalized and the levels of payment expanded, but these changes have come after the closure of this study of rural primary care programs.

The general economic climate for rural America during the 1980s was one of impending crisis. Bad weather in farm-dependent states, the reversal of the urban-to-rural migration pattern, and a general softening of the economy left many rural communities in desperate straits by the end of the decade. These trends were reflected in the fiscal positions of primary care programs and physicians' practices throughout the rural portion of the United States (National Rural Health Association, 1988b).

Service Areas and Populations Served

Demographic and Socioeconomic Characteristics of Service Area Populations

The programs were asked several questions concerning the makeup of their service populations. The communities in which the 40 rural primary care programs were located experienced changes in several socioeconomic factors between 1980 and 1989. For example, the proportion of families in the programs' service areas living below the poverty line increased from 24 to 36 percent over the decade. Infant mortality rates dropped on average from 14.4 to 11.1 in the counties where these programs were located.

There were also changes in the insurance coverage of clinic users. The percentage of clinic users with no insurance coverage increased from 34 to 44 percent; the proportion of those with Medicaid coverage remained at 19 percent, and the percentage of users with Medicare demonstrated a decrease from 19 to 14 percent.

The racial composition of the service areas for each program's principal site showed a slight trend over the period 1980–1989 toward larger proportions of minorities, with the percentage of users that were white but not Hispanic decreasing from 63 to 57 percent, that of Hispanics increasing from 16 to 17 percent, and that of blacks increasing slightly from 16 to 18 percent of medical users. The proportion of American Indians and other groups increased from 5 to 8 percent of site users.

The service area population from which the programs' principal sites drew their patients increased, on average, from 13,705 to 15,398 in the period 1980–1989; this potential increase in demand for services was not met by increased resources and health care staff levels, as will be shown in subsequent sections.

Other Medical Resources Available in Program Service Areas

Clinic patients and staff traveled on average twenty-five minutes to the nearest hospital according to the 1989 responses; the range in travel times was from zero minutes to two hours. Of the hospitals in the study site communities most used by program patients in 1981, all remained open during the decade except for one, a thirty-bed hospital in a western state (program #10828). Access to hospital services does not appear to have decreased for the service population of this program, since the program is now administered by a hospital fifteen miles away. In addition, a ninety-eight-bed hospital just seventeen miles from a health center in a southwestern state (program #10865) was opened during the decade, replacing a larger hospital forty-five minutes away as the facility most used by clinic patients. The nearest hospital to the principal site was not always used by most clinic patients in all programs. For example, poor patients of a program located in a particularly economically depressed state, where Medicaid eligibility is very restricted (program #10635), are required to go to one of the state charity hospitals over fifty miles away from the clinic site, and can be admitted only by state M.D.s from the medical schools, despite there being a small hospital located within one block of the clinic. In general, however, it appears that programs developed a somewhat closer relationship with their area hospitals through the decade. Two programs that were independently governed in 1981 are now administered by local hospitals. In 1981, out of thirty-five reporting programs, the median percentage of program patients needing hospitalization that were admitted by site staff was 68 percent. This figure increased to a median of 88 percent in 1989 for twenty-seven programs that reported data. This increase could be a product of more program physicians receiving hospital privileges over the timespan. Thirty-four percent of questionnaire respondents (thirteen out of thirty-eight) reported in 1981 that securing hospital privileges was a moderate to severe problem; this figure dropped to 13 percent (four out of thirty-one) in 1989. Health services offered by other organizations in program communities will be described later in this chapter.

Other Providers in the Service Areas

On average, the number of other primary care providers in the programs' service areas was over two times higher in 1989 than in 1980, increasing from 4.2 to 11 providers in the communities for which data were available. In 1980 there were no other nonprogram primary care providers in eighteen program service areas; in 1989, only six of the programs reported that they were the sole providers in the community. Considering population growth along with growth in physician supply, the average physician-to-population ratio of the counties in which the programs are located increased from 8 per 1,000 to 9 per 1,000 residents. This characteristic of the communities puts them in contrast to other rural areas in the United States.

In 1981, twelve out of thirty-eight (32 percent) of the programs responding reported that one or more of the other health care providers in the programs' service areas refused to serve specific groups of patients. Of these twelve, nine communities had providers who turned away Medicaid patients, eight refused service to the medically indigent, six denied health care to migrants, and five refused service to minorities. This situation apparently did not improve over the decade, as evidenced by twelve of the thirty-one programs responding to this question in 1989 (39 percent) reporting that other providers in their communities refused service to particular groups of patients. However, although eleven of these twelve communities had providers in 1989 who refused service to the medically indigent and seven, to Medicaid patients, discrimination against migrants was found in only one service area and none of the questionnaire respondents in 1989 reported denial of health services to minorities. Opposition to the programs by local providers in the communities, as reported by question-naire respondents, dropped slightly during the decade, with 40 percent (fifteen out of thirty-seven respondents) having either a moderate or severe problem in 1981 and 32 percent (ten out of thirty-one operating programs) experiencing this level of opposi-tion in 1989. An example of opposition faced in 1981 by one program was the objection of a local medical society to federal intervention in health care in the community (program #22335). This situation still held in 1989, but the program had won the acceptance of area residents and managed to increase its level of productivity in delivering health services to the community dur-ing the decade.

Program Operation

Changes in Organization

Of the forty subsidized rural primary care programs operating in 1980, thirty-three continue in some form as primary health care centers, publicly supported or nonprofit. Four merged into or were subsumed under other organizations and five changed into private practices. Only two have completely closed during the decade. Of these two, one program dissolved because the number of physicians in the area increased, and the organization was not considered necessary to serve the community. That program (#10786) was based in a small hospital in an economically stable community. Informants who had left the site felt that the program served well as a temporary solution to a local physician shortage. The other closed program has not been replaced by a private practice or by another subsidized primary care organization in the community.

Four programs merged with other similar subsidized programs. One program (#10401), in a southeastern state, was once an auton-omous CHC with a series of its own satellites and a well-defined local, rural constituency. However, it lost out in a struggle with an urban CHC thirty-five miles distant when funding was cut in 1983; and the merger with the urban program was not completely welcomed by the staff and board of the rural program. A similar pattern of merger was seen in another CHC (#10395) in the southeast that was absorbed into a metropolitan CHC forty-seven miles distant. The smaller, rural program was having difficulty in keeping its board unified, and staff turnover and management problems led to its merger into the more stable urban system. Two other single-site programs (#10407 and #20205) merged into larger programs that served rural areas as well as large towns in nonmetropolitan counties. Each of the latter two programs was unable to maintain patient volume sufficient to support independent management capacity.

Five programs went through a transition from being publicly subsidized to operating as private practices; these practices remained in the same location, serve the same general service population as the previous program, and, in most cases, retained some of the same personnel that were there in 1980. The five programs were in medium-sized rural communities in counties adjacent to metropolitan counties, and their transition from public funding to private operation could have been predicted at the time of the original site visits.

Twenty-nine of the forty continued providing services to their communities in the same general organizational form from 1980 to 1989. Of these twenty-nine, four showed a reduction in services, measured by a reduction in staff, users or encounters by greater than half, three increased function by over 50 percent, and twenty-two continued at the same level of function.

It is notable that all but two of the programs (95 percent) have managed to remain in operation over a period when there have been marked fluctuations in availability of outside funding. The decreased availability to these programs of most types of government funds will be detailed in a subsequent section of this chapter. Many of the programs appear to have struggled throughout the decade either to remain operating or to maintain the same level of services provided in 1980, and have adopted different survival strategies. Some programs have made a priority of avoiding dependence on federal funds, instead relying on subsidy from local governments, private foundation support, and community fund raising. A strategy mentioned earlier, adjusting to cuts in outside funding by transformation into a private practice arrangement, was employed by five programs. There is variation among these five in the degree to which they continue to provide primary health care services to their communities. However, these conversions to self-support may be viewed as successes, in general, since most of these programs continue to provide services in areas where there are deficits in supply of other primary health care personnel. Most of these transformed programs have survived without outside funds for over five years without reducing staff significantly.

For many, it appears that the dedication and continuity provided by program staff has been a key factor in the survival and prosperity of the practices. This can also be seen in programs where reduction in outside funds has led to reduction in staff and services. For example, two programs in the sample have suffered losses of federal CHC funds, and operate currently with fewer services and reduced hours from their 1980 level of activity. These programs (#10279 and #10865) were able to tighten their budgets while at the same time striving to continue to provide needed services to their service populations. One of these has become essentially self-sufficient; liberal Medicaid reimbursement combined with a low program budget and the continuing efforts of two staff members who have been at the clinic through the decade are cited as reasons for the survival of this clinic. Four programs have increased services to their service populations over the decade, adding additional sites, providers, and services.

In the National Evaluation of Rural Primary Care Programs, undertaken over ten years ago and described in the opening of this chapter, rural primary care programs were classified and selected for study according to a typology of practice organizations. This typology has been described in depth elsewhere (Sheps et al., 1983). At the outset of the evaluation, the programs selected for site visits were restricted to three forms: (1) comprehensive health centers, (2) organized group practices, and (3) primary care centers. Of the forty sites, five of the CHCs, two of the OGPs, and six of the PCCs changed form, according to the original algorithm. Outreach services, a defining characteristic of the CHC organizational form, were cut from many programs, therefore prohibiting these programs from being defined as CHCs. The proportion of OGPs increased; these programs have fewer primary care providers than CHCs, no community outreach services are provided, and the providers are paid on the basis of productivity. The percentage of PCCs decreased, possibly signaling a trend away from these smaller programs and a drop in the distribution of midlevel providers in rural areas. Another potential interpretation focuses on the community structure of the PCCs, which were seen to be more closely integrated into local community infrastructures where the development and maintenance of these programs is stimulated and/or subsidized through local community involvement; that local investment may have faltered over time or been replaced by external funding. Institutional extension practices are controlled by an external organization, such as a hospital; two programs evolved into this form over the decade, both being turned into ambulatory outposts of medium-sized hospitals.

One important modification of program structure and operation was undertaken by a multisite program located in the south. This program (#10310) was a comprehensive health center funded by the Section 330 (CHC) and 329 (MHC) programs. The communities that the program served were very poor and the patient population was dominated by migrant and seasonal workers. The program with its four sites was constantly in need of primary care providers and usually was staffed by NHSC scholarship recipients or foreign medical graduates who were part of the large immigrant population in the state. At the time of the initial site visit, the program was recruiting in much the same way as other primary care delivery systems, through advertising to and direct mail contact with new medical graduates and through the efforts of the state primary care association. In 1981 and 1982, the development of a new osteopathic medical school in a metropolitan area eighty miles to the southeast provided a unique opportunity for the program. That osteopathic school included as one of its primary missions the training of osteopathic physicians for the host state who would be well prepared to deliver care to the elderly, indigents, and rural communities. As the founders of the school began to develop their curricula they decided that each undergraduate student should have a three-month rural clerkship in an underserved area. The school began recruiting clinical sites for this requirement and the target program provided four such sites. The program was now affiliated directly with a medical school, and the staff at the clinic sites were able to interact with the regular faculty of the school, who oversaw the clerkships, as well as make use of the skills of the students and residents who also were placed in the program sites. This program has been in place since 1984 and the providers and administrator of the program all agree that it has contributed to the quality of care the program is able to deliver and provided an additional recruiting advantage.

This rurally based training program is a unique example of a regularized system of training in underserved areas; it is unique because the rotating clerkships are required and emphasized, because there is a linked didactic requirement in rural and minority medicine in the first two years of medical school, and because the medical school is committed to the continued viability of the rural primary care programs and makes an effort to place its graduates in the underserved sites. The osteopathic medical school also makes use of health department facilities and mental health clinics in other community-based programs for placing medical students and residents. This unified approach to health care gives students a more holistic view of community medicine and the needs of the underserved populations. This program may be considered a model for the linkage of training and service delivery aimed at alleviating the problem of medical underservice in rural America.

Trends in Services Offered by the Programs

Programs generally seem to have adjusted to changes in sources of funding and possibly to decreased community involvement by cutting a number of services and maintaining or increasing a few selected services.

Of the nine services listed in table 9.1, it is evident that the most marked changes during the period 1981–1989 are found in the decrease in provision of outreach services and the increase in provision of well child care. In addition, although the number of programs offering family planning services decreased during the decade, these services remain in the greatest proportion of the programs. Comparing trends from 1981 to 1989, the decrease in outreach, transportation, and family planning services provided by programs is apparently not being compensated for elsewhere in program communities.

Although there was a decrease in social services provided elsewhere in program communities, the programs themselves collectively increased their emphasis on these services. The largest increase was seen in availability of well child care in the rural primary care programs, although there was a concomitant decrease in this service in the communities.

Table 9.1. Trends in Services Provided by the Programs

Service	Programs providing service in 1981		Programs providing service in 1989		Change (%)
	No.	Percent	No.	Percent	
Outreach services	30	83	13	36	–47
Transportation	30	83	16	44	–39
Prenatal care	33	92	23	64	–28
Mental health care	15	42	10	28	–14
Family planning	35	97	30	83	–14
Dental care	13	36	13	36	0
Home care	9	25	11	31	6
Social services	10	28	15	42	14
Well child care	7	19	28	78	59

Note: Information available for thirty-six programs.

From 1981 to 1989, the principal delivery sites of the programs increased the availability of on-site blood sodium and potassium testing, with from 22 percent to 70 percent providing this clinical service. The provision of chest X-rays at the principal sites did not change appreciably, with 62 percent of the sites offering this diagnostic test in 1981 and 61 percent in 1989. A greater percentage of the operating programs in 1989 had licensed pharmacies than did those in 1981 (47 percent compared to 32 percent).

Policy Decisions: Trends

The National Evaluation attempted to examine the effects of different patterns of decision-making on the stability and impacts of the programs. The key respondents were asked which of five classes of decision-makers in the program—medical director, other provider, administrator, governing board, or external agency—had the most influence on ten strategic decisions. The original evaluation was primarily concerned with the power and influence of the board on program operation; heavy board involvement in decision-making was related to lower financial stability but greater impacts on access. In the 1989 follow-up, program informants were asked who had final authority concerning six strategic decisions.

In 1981, the administrators of the thirty-seven programs for which data were available had final authority on an average of 42 percent of the decisions, the board members were responsible for a total of 26 percent of the policy decisions, the medical directors made 31 percent of the decisions, external institutions made 5 percent, and 5 percent of decisions were made jointly. In 1989, from data available for thirty-two programs, the percentage of total final decisions that were made by administrators alone increased to 48 percent; the board's control of decisions declined to 14 percent, and the medical directors' decreased to 19 percent.

In contrast to programs in 1981, 15 percent of policy decisions made in 1989 were said to be decisions made in conjunction by two or more of the above-mentioned decision-makers.

Programs Developed in Comparison Communities

Eight comparison communities were surveyed in 1981; these were chosen from a universe of approximately sixty communities across the United States that were about to initiate a subsidized rural health clinic or had applied for support for a primary care clinic. The sample was selected to compare the impact of the programs on community access as measured by surveys of community residents. Samples of residents from each of these communities were surveyed for information describing their health status and use of health services.

Of the eight communities, four have developed rural primary care programs in the period since 1981. Follow-up questionnaires, similar to the mailed survey instrument that was sent to the forty rural sites, were sent to these four programs in 1989; a full set of information was obtained from three of the programs. Three communities received federal funding for their programs. Two of these three can be classified as PCCs according to the typology discussed previously; each has exactly one full-time M.D. and each has a degree of community involvement. Information was not available to classify the third funded program. The fourth center can be classified as an institutional extension hospital satellite; this clinic is administered by a hospital sixty miles away, does not receive any outside funding, and serves an isolated rural population without other sources of primary care in the immediate area. In this case the distance of the people from available care appears to have been more influential than the level of poverty of the population in development of the clinic.

Finance

Among the thirty-three programs that continued as one of the publicly supported or nonprofit primary health care centers, the proportion of their total income derived from patient revenues decreased from 60 to 54 percent, whereas the portion of patient income from hospital revenues increased from 8 to 10 percent. The proportion of billed charges actually collected by the programs rose from 68 to 81 percent, even though the percentage of patients covered by any type of insurance dropped significantly over the decade. The ability of the programs to raise their total collection rates is somewhat surprising, given the fact that in 1981 reimbursement from Medicaid was reported to be a moderate to severe problem in 47 percent (eighteen out of thirty-eight responding) of the programs, whereas this problem was reported in 68 percent (twenty-one out of thirty-one responding) in 1989. Nineteen percent of clinic users were covered by Medicaid in both 1981 and 1989. Program staff may have developed more efficient means of managing their centers to deal with decreasing ability of clinic users to pay for services. Analysis of financial data from the 1980–1981 surveys found that there is a strong relationship between smaller program size and higher collection rates (University of North Carolina Health Services Research Center, 1983). However, medical encounters at the principal sites also increased by approximately 28 percent (from 12,474 to 15,987 in the programs for which data were available) while the collection rate rose, indicating increased productivity.

Trends in the sources of outside funding for the programs showed some maturation of the programs. Although federal funding opportunities generally decreased, with the exception of an increased percentage of programs receiving CHC funds, programs received more support from state governments. Seven programs were completely self-supporting in 1989, whereas all had been subsidized to some extent in 1981.

In 1981, thirty of the thirty-seven programs (81%) for which data were available responded that their programs used a sliding fee scale based on income. This is comparable to the 74 percent (twenty-five out of thirty-four) of the operating programs for which data were available that used a sliding fee scale in 1989. There was a wide range in percentage of patients accepted on a sliding fee basis, from 1 to 99 percent, averaging 49 percent of patients in 1989, compared to 46 percent in 1981.

Sliding fee proportions were strongly associated with financial self-sufficiency in the original study. The higher proportion in the 1989 data would, based on the earlier data, indicate greater stress on the programs. The high percentage of survivors suggests that the application of the sliding fee may have been altered to reduce its effect on the fiscal position of the programs, or that programs have been able to replace revenue lost through the reduced fee arrangements.

The programs were very responsive to environmental stresses and opportunities, and this was reflected in their ability to adapt constructively. Each of the programs included in the sample in this study felt some degree of stress over the ten-year period in which they were studied. The two that closed were in communities that were able to replace their health care capacity through means other than a clinic, center, or program, subsidized or not. Three programs were able to increase their level of providers, medical users, or encounters by greater than 100 percent; two of these were CHCs and one was an OGP in 1989 (#10283, #10436, and #22335). These programs, of which two were in southern states and one in a western state, received greater amounts of federal and state funds in 1989 than in 1981, generally had higher than average percentages of their service populations living below the poverty level, had higher percentages of minorities in their service populations, and in most cases had relatively high collection rates. These programs were able to recruit a number of new providers over the time period, even though only one received NHSC funds in 1989.

Summary, Conclusions, Implications

Primary care programs represent a persisting and effective mechanism to increase the availability of appropriate health care services to smaller rural communities. In the sample examined in this chapter, the centers and programs also provided needed services in larger rural communities where the existing providers were unwilling or unable to serve certain segments of the local population. The ability of these programs to survive is testament to the original intentions of the legislators, agency officials, and program leaders who initiated the many interventions that led to their opening. The programs have changed in their commitment to community input as the nature of community governance has caused some problems. Still, the programs see their role as community-oriented if not community-responsive despite pressures to cast them into the mold of the private ambulatory practice of medicine.

The programs that we studied have been able to change in ways that might not have been predicted in 1978 or earlier. The pattern of merger we observed in several programs reflected a change in the politics of CHCs, where more urban centers were able to dominate smaller, rural programs. This change holds important and portentous promise for rural programs; they may find themselves losing their rural identity and autonomy if there is a movement toward the "rationalization" or regionalization of primary care programs driven by political or financial interests. The merger of programs into hospitals may point toward either a rural- or an urban-oriented system of regionalization of services. There are rural hospitals that might well ally themselves with rural primary care centers to strengthen both organizations, the former by developing a referral base, the latter by providing continuity of care and reinforcing the professional environment for the providers. On the other hand, the rural centers may become simple outposts for referrals to more urban hospitals. Again, there is the threat that the rural communities will lose some measure of control over their clinical resources. Each of these two patterns was observed in the study.

The dominant pressures of the 1980s on these programs may have caused them to adjust their organizational structures and procedures to cope with a changing and tightening fiscal environment. They were, in a sense, learning to compete. Today, that preoccupation with income may be replaced with an overriding concern with staffing as the NHSC ceases to be an option for the relatively easy recruitment of providers. There is evidence that the pattern of turnover exhibited during the 1980s in these programs is one that can allow for rural primary care organizations to continue to meet their clinical and financial needs while managing a reasonable level of personnel change. We do not know, however, if that pattern can be sustained without the corps and if longer vacancies and more difficult recruitment pressures hold. Can these programs survive under these constraints? We were not able to predict this but certainly feel that staffing will be the issue of the 1990s.

Another characteristic of many of the programs may also point to future solutions for the persistent maldistribution of health care resources that rural people experience. Several of the programs studied have been able to innovate in strikingly new directions. The example of the osteopathic medical school connection with one of the CHCs supports this observation. That program has been able to improve care and stabilize its staffing through an ambitious but feasible arrangement that trades some efficiency for stability. Other programs have been able to develop new linkages as other rural organizations try to combine the resources needed to survive. If staffing is to be the problem of the 1990s, then organizational innovation is the potential solution to most of the other problems of rural primary care delivery.

Chapter 10

Consumer Choice and the National Rural Hospital Crisis

GORDON H. DeFRIESE, GLENN WILSON,
THOMAS C. RICKETTS, AND
LYNN WHITENER

Whether in terms of size, the characteristics of their client populations, the competition they face from other health care providers, or their remote location, rural hospitals in the United States operate at a disadvantage compared to metropolitan hospitals. Between 1980 and 1987, 519 U.S. hospitals closed or ceased to provide inpatient medical care. Of those hospitals that closed during this seven-year period, 364 were community hospitals. Rural hospitals accounted for 163 (45 percent) of these community hospital closures. Between 1983 and 1987, more than 70 percent of the rural hospitals that closed were ones with fewer than fifty beds (American Hospital Association, 1989; Mullner and McNeil, 1986).

These institutions occupy particularly important positions in the communities they serve. Not only are they the focal points of local health care delivery systems, but they also serve as an important aspect of the physician recruitment effort. Moreover, these institutions serve to provide a source of civic self-esteem and are an important aspect of the local economy. The jobs they create and the steady flow of public and private funds they bring in as payment for services act to stimulate local business and employment prospects. The decision to close or convert these facilities to other uses is a critical decision having broad implications for almost every aspect of the social and economic situation facing these rural communities (Christianson and Faulkner, 1981).

The situation faced by rural hospitals is complicated by the burdens of an aging rural population, a disproportionate share of the nation's families and individuals living in poverty, widespread unemployment or underemployment, a population that is inadequately insured with regard to health care, a declining population base, and extreme shortages of needed health care personnel in every category (Melcher, 1988).

It is the conventional wisdom that the federal Medicare program has had much to do with the current financial situation facing rural hospitals in this country. The increasing dependence of these institutions on revenues generated through service to an aging population insured through the Medicare program means that even slight changes in the provisions of this federal program can have enormous consequences for all aspects of rural hospitals' operational stability and quality of care. The Medicare program differentially reimburses rural hospitals for the care they provide and the program's payment procedures act to the disadvantage of these, usually small, facilities (Bean, 1988). The initial enactment of differential Medicare price schedules between urban and rural hospitals under the Prospective Payment System (PPS), and the slow transition to national rates of payment, have acted to create serious cash flow problems for these rural hospitals. Moreover, the Medicare program calculates rates of payment on the basis of average costs at each institution. The fact that some of these rural hospitals serve such restricted numbers of patients means that they cannot take advantage of the "law of large numbers," which enables larger hospitals to offset the effects of expensive outlier cases within their caseloads.

Twenty-five percent of all rural hospitals had negative margins of −9.1 percent or worse (Prospective Payment Assessment Commission, 1988); 10 percent of those hospitals with less than 50 beds had negative margins of −44.7 percent or worse (Gilligan et al., 1988).

Caution should be exercised to avoid the implication that Medicare and Medicaid are the sole reason, or are largely responsible, for the plight of rural hospitals in this country. A review of hospital statistics published by the American Hospital Association has shown that for many years prior to the inauguration of PPS (under diagnostic-related groups methods), bed-days of care for hospitals of less than fifty beds dropped by 35 percent from 1973 to 1983. Hospitals of fifty to ninety-nine beds increased bed-days of care by 10 percent during the same period. The problems of small rural hospitals are a *long-term* issue that may have been *made worse* by Medicare reimbursement.

There are other factors to consider. Rural communities throughout the nation are in a state of general social and economic decline. With the exodus of population it is possible that the resources to support the infrastructure of health and human services simply do not exist. The hospital crisis may be merely a symptom of a much larger problem, one that the Medicare program, through any attempt to readjust the basis of its payment formula, cannot address. Many have pointed to the fact that, without the physicians to provide primary care and then to produce the demand for in-hospital patient care and ancillary services, hospitals cannot exist in these communities. With only 53 physicians per 100,000 people in rural areas (as compared with 160 per 100,000 in urban areas), the physician shortage is dramatic and increasingly apparent. We have not seen really effective means of developing what might be called "systems" of health care for rural communities. A solution to the problem of the rural hospital may require a multifaceted approach involving the full spectrum of health and medical care services (Amundson and Rosenblatt, 1988). This strategy may mean that the surviving rural hospital of the future will find itself involved in the provision of a different array of services than at present, thus occupying a very different niche in the overall ecology of health care serving rural populations.

An important factor to consider is the nature of local *primary* health care services. It is through and in conjunction with primary health care providers that rural hospitals come to play whatever role they do in the total care of defined populations. If we are to understand the future of the rural hospital, we must understand the need and demand for primary health care services among rural community residents. The relationship between hospitals and primary care providers is clearly mutually influential (McLaughlin et al., 1985).

The national policy debate surrounding the rural hospital is one in which clear decisional direction presents a formidable analytical task. This is made all the more difficult because of the absence of widely accepted *goals* for health care policy development. To some, the goal in the rural health arena should be to give every person who resides in a nonmetropolitan area the same access to every level of health care as any resident of a metropolitan community. Although there are few who would actually see this goal as within the realm of possibility, the advocacy of this approach as a general (explicit or implicit) guide to policy development puts serious constraints on what can be done to address these issues. Others maintain that rural communities, especially those that are most remote, must be guaranteed direct and immediate access to certain fundamental types of health care, but that access to the full spectrum of health care can only be given through triage and referral to larger health care facilities in metropolitan areas.

Recent, and as yet unpublished, data from a study by Health Economics Research, Inc., and Abt Associates, Inc., for the Health Care Financing Administration identified twenty-five rural hospital closures between 1980 and 1986 in each of which the hospital was the sole (i.e., "monopoly") acute care facility in the county (Hendricks, 1989). The average number of beds in these hospitals was twenty-four, compared with seventy-seven for all rural hospitals. During the study period (1980–1986), admissions fell by an average of 18 percent between 1980 and the year the hospital closed.

The surprising finding in this study relevant to the present inquiry is that "despite these hospital closures, few of these counties appear to be unserved. Half of the counties that lost their sole inpatient facility were adjacent to a Metropolitan Statistical Area." Though the residents of these communities must now travel further to seek inpatient care, there is a considerable difference between being *unserved* and a condition of *underservice*, as defined by some criterion of distance to the nearest health care facility. Given the fact that most of those institutions that closed were ones in close proximity to metropolitan areas and had experienced low levels of occupancy for many years prior to their closure, perhaps the health care consumers in these communities have in effect defined, for many years, the conditions of organizational survival. They have, as is often said, *voted with their feet.*

To understand this set of circumstances more fully—to understand the policy options of greatest public benefit and preference—we need to know more about the consumer's view of these facilities, their presumed utility in time of need, and consumer preferences with respect to a whole range of health care options and choices.

Public Policy Attention to Rural Hospitals

The nature of this inquiry is both timely and important. First of all, there is at present a rising concern in the public and private health care sectors, as well as within Congress, over the special problem of rural communities with regard to basic health care services (Hewitt, 1989). The burden of rural hospital failure has not been entirely borne by not-for-profit community general hospitals. A recent study completed by Mullner et al. (1988) shows that, even though only 8.2 percent of rural community hospitals are owned by for-profit concerns, 24.5 percent of those rural community hospitals that closed between 1980 and 1987 were for-profit facilities. Not-for-profit, nongovernmental facilities accounted for 43.5 percent of closures, while state and local governmental facilities accounted for 32 percent. Hence, this is a problem of broad significance and is not limited to only one type of facility ownership.

Several solutions have been proposed to the financial problems of rural hospitals. Among these proposals are options such as these:

- Eliminating the disparity between urban and rural hospitals in rates of payment under Medicare PPS
- Creating a single national rate for hospital compensation
- Assisting rural hospitals with the conversion of some or all of their current capacity to uses other than acute inpatient care
- Allowing some or all rural hospitals to go back on a cost-based reimbursement formula for a limited period of time until PPS can be better adjusted for urban hospitals, then redesigning a form of PPS suitable for rural hospitals
- Giving rural hospitals a higher rate of increase than urban hospitals in their PPS rates (an option that has been proposed many times in the past)

What is absent from these proposals is any real information about the patterns of hospital services utilization or consumer preferences for hospital services among persons who live in the communities being served by these facilities. Moreover, there is a lack of cohesiveness in the framework of policy development in this area and a failure to take explicit account of the way in which primary health care services are utilized and how patterns of use for that level of care influence the need and demand for in-hospital care.

The literature on the current fiscal and administrative situation facing the nation's rural hospitals is neither extensive nor especially relevant to the question of consumer preferences with regard to acute hospital care among the residents of rural communities. The most comprehensive reviews of the literature on rural hospitals have been prepared by Moscovice and Rosenblatt (Moscovice and Rosenblatt, 1982b; 1985a,b; Moscovice, 1989). Moscovice (1989) has pointed out that there has not been extensive research on the performance of rural hospitals, and that most of the research that does exist has focused on descriptive case studies, which have been limited in their generalizability by the diversity of rural hospitals. It is apparent from these several reviews that practically no attention has thus far been paid to the behavior of rural health care consumers with regard to inpatient, acute hospital care.

Before examining those studies that have actually measured consumer preferences in the rural hospital care arena, we first describe conventional research on the factors that pose the greatest risk of hospital closure and the way in which the services utilization behavior of rural residents has been imputed as an underlying causal variable.

Studies of Hospital Closure

The majority of studies of hospital closure have thus far attempted to identify those structural or environmental factors that might account for (or predict) the closure of hospitals. Three studies seem to occupy the more prominent places in this literature.

The first of these is the study by Mayer et al. (1987), a case-control study of 148 rural hospitals that closed between 1970 and 1980 matched with 310 comparable hospitals that remained open during the same period. This study found that closed and open hospitals differed with respect to internal (structural) characteristics and attributes of their local geographic areas. Among the factors found to differentiate between those hospitals that closed and those that remained open were ownership status, occupancy rate, competitive beds within the county, scope of service, and county population change during the preceding decade.

Similar findings emerged from a second case-control study of 161 rural hospitals that closed between 1980 and 1987 by Mullner et al. (1989) In this study, closed hospitals were matched (1 : 3) with 483 rural hospitals that remained open. Four variables seemed to relate in a positive (direct) way to the risk of hospital closure: (1) for-profit ownership, (2) nongovernmental, not-for-profit ownership, (3) presence of a skilled nursing or other long-term care unit in the county, and (4) the number of other hospitals in the county. Three variables seemed to have negative (indirect) relationships with hospital closure: (1) JCAHCO accreditation, (2) number of facilities and services offered by the hospital, and (3) membership of the hospital in a multihospital system. This study proposed a number of policy considerations intended to improve the financial advantage of small, rural hospitals, especially recommendations having to do with the way such hospitals were paid for services to Medicare beneficiaries.

The third study of some importance is one by Morrisey et al. (1989) that explored the structural determinants of rural hospital performance. This paper provides a good discussion of basic issues, including empirical approaches, related to market area research and policy analysis in health care. The authors apply these basic concepts and methods of market area definition to the situation of single-hospital counties in Nebraska. There were twenty-seven single-hospital counties in Nebraska at the time of the study. In this study, each hospital on average received only 54 percent of its discharges from residents of the county in which it was located (with a range of 18 to 98 percent). On the other hand, 72 percent of all hospital discharges for persons with residences in the focal county were discharges from the focal hospital (with a range of 47 to 93 percent).

It appeared from a case-mix analysis performed as part of this study that there are some hospital products (e.g., high-technology acute care) that are not provided by small rural hospitals. Rural residents admitted from urban hospitals tended to be more severely ill. This study suggests that the market area for certain kinds of hospital services may differ considerably from one type of service to another. Consumers' patterns of demand, and the service offerings of rural hospitals, reflect a profile of care that characterizes the special nature of rural hospitals vis-à-vis their principal constituency.

This finding is similar to that from the study by Hogan (1988) in which it was found that individuals in rural areas of New York state who traveled beyond their own county or the counties adjacent to their own in search of hospital care were persons with a higher case-mix index (i.e., were more severely ill), but were less likely to be older than seventy-five years of age.

These findings suggest that, if we are to move beyond a structural analysis of factors associated with the characteristics of hospitals and their geographic areas in the study of rural hospital prospects for long-term survival, we must begin to focus on the characteristics of patient conditions, the acuity with which patients and their families associate these conditions, and the perception these consumers have of the technological requirements of a given condition.

Medical Geographic Studies of Patient Outshopping Behavior

One of the most important bodies of social science literature related to the questions addressed in this review has emerged from the field of medical geography, where there has been a long-standing interest in health care utilization behavior. (We draw in this section on an unpublished review of medical geographic studies of the rural hospital problem prepared for the North Carolina Rural Health Research Program in 1989 by Kathryn Byrnes of the University of North Carolina at Chapel Hill Department of Geography.) The most widely accepted theory in medical geography holds that, *ceteris paribus,* consumers will use those services located nearest to them in times of need. Christaller's central place theory assumes that consumers will travel only as far as necessary to obtain a desired service or good (Christaller, 1933). Patterns of use different from this nearest-place model are defined as aberrant utilization behavior.

This theoretical perspective has given rise to the concept of distance decay, whereby medical geographers have postulated that social (and economic) interactions over space decline with increasing distance. That is, rates of use (or rates of preference) for particular goods or services fall off with increasing distance to them (Moseley, 1979). Using the notion of intervening opportunities advanced by the famous sociologist Samuel A. Stouffer, geographers have also focused their research on the effects of alternative sources of particular goods and services on consumer preferences. Research in this direction related to hospital and medical care has found that, as the distance between the nearest source of such services and an alternative *decreases,* the proportion of consumers who are willing to consider (and who actually use) an alternative facility or provider *increases* (Weiss et al., 1971). Hence, the tendency for out-of-area shopping (or "outshopping") for goods and services is inversely related to the distance to alternate sources for those goods and services.

This research has led to the concept of the *hierarchial structure* of health care services and facilities (Shannon et al., 1969). It is argued by contemporary medical geographers who have studied patterns of health services consumer behavior that, though there is a distance beyond which patients are unable and unwilling to travel in search of needed health care (Bashshur et al., 1971), the effect/relevance of distance varies with the services or products for which the need exists (Roghmann and Zastowny, 1979). Research in this field has shown that health care consumers will travel farther the more *specialized* they consider the services required (Kane, 1969), the more *urgent or acute* they consider the need to be (Roghmann and Zastowny, 1979), or the more *sophisticated* they have defined one source to be than another (Magnusson, 1980).

Hence, the field of medical geography leads us to define the hospital as a provider of a *bundle* of more or less distinct services, each of which has its own distinctive catchment area and associated patient/consumer travel patterns. The willingness of consumers of health care services to consider an outshopping strategy of access to these services is likely to vary among among distinct categories of services. Thus, it is important to make a distinction among several sets of services of interest to consumers in any attempt to define the geographic patterns of hospital service use.

Studies of Hospital Consumer Behavior

Though there has been a general interest in the health services research and medical sociological literature for more than a decade in the study of patterns of shopping for physician care (Gray and Cartwright, 1953; Kasteler et al., 1976), there has been relatively little research on the patterns of shopping for hospital care. The study of intermarket patronage among consumers of any type of product has been an issue of considerable interest in the marketing field for many years. The notion of the outshopper (Hawes and Lumpkin, 1984) is one of importance to the understanding of patterns of use of hospital care by rural community residents.

Three studies attempt to explain patterns of consumer use of rural hospital services and facilities. The first of these is by Hart, Rosenblatt, and Amundson and involves the survey by mailed questionnaire of the total population of households in the service areas of six hospitals selected from the states of Washington, Alaska, Montana, and Idaho as part of the Rural Hospital Project of the University of Washington at Seattle (Hart et al., 1989; Amundson and Rosenblatt, 1988). Response rates ranged from 24 to 36 percent. Overall, there were more than 6,000 household responses.

These surveys attempted to measure hospital service utilization, satisfaction with local hospital facilities and services, and feelings about local physicians. The results of these surveys indicated that older residents of these communities, and those with better insurance coverage, tended to be more satisfied with the quality of hospital care available to them in their local communities than younger and less well-insured residents. Second, satisfaction with the local hospital seemed to correlate highly with perceptions about the hospital's billing practices and feelings about the emergency room and the way it operated. Respondents seemed to reflect feelings and attitudes about the local hospital that were similar to, or dependent upon, their feelings and attitudes about the quality of local physician services.

It was recommended that one way in which a local community could increase the market share of a local rural hospital would be to increase the number of local residents with personal physicians resident in the community. Because of the nature and mix of medical needs in any given population, this would mean that the mix of local physician specialties would have to coincide with these medical needs and demands. In addition, the report recommended that the local hospital strengthen the capacity and responsiveness of its emergency room in order for its clientele to evaluate the hospital's overall quality at a higher level.

The second study emerged from the W. K. Kellogg Foundation–supported demonstration projects in Colorado, Montana, and North Dakota called Affordable Rural Coalitions for Health (ARCH) (Ludtke et al., 1989). In this project, local coalitions of civic and health sector leaders came together to consider a broad range of health program and service needs, among them the future of the local hospital facilities. Part of this project in the nine sites studied, all of which had hospitals, involved a mailed questionnaire to random samples of residents of each of these communities as part of the ARCH planning process. A total aggregate sample of 1,848 respondents (with a response rate of 43.6 percent) was obtained.

The study analyzed patterns of consumer outshopping for hospital and medical care in these communities, which ranged in population size from 935 to 15,502. Several categories of explanatory variables were included in the survey questionnaires: *predisposing factors* (individual characteristics, such as beliefs and attitudes regarding the value of health or respondent education, occupation, income, race, age, sex, or length of residence in the community); *enabling factors* (e.g., financial resources, insurance coverage, costs of services, and physical access to care); *medical need* (health status and health perceptions; disability days and days of restricted activity); and *attitudinal factors* (such as those toward locally available services, consumer preferences, and provider selection variables, e.g., rating of local community as a place to live and work). The latter group of variables proved to be much more important as a predictor of outshopping than might have been expected. The "image" of the local community among community residents had much to do with whether these families were likely to shop for medical and hospital care in their own communities or go outside for such services. The relative importance of attitude variables in relation to medical need and enabling variables indicated the importance of measuring the way in which a local community may be rated, in a general way, in any attempt to understand patterns of health care shopping behavior.

In a third study, Bindman undertook to survey 219 former patients of a community hospital in California that closed, and a comparison sample of 195 residents of a nearby community where a similar type of hospital stayed open (Bindman, 1989). In both communities surveys were conducted at baseline (shortly before the closure of the focal hospital was announced) and one year after closure. Ninety percent of patients at both hospitals could be reinterviewed at one year. Questionnaire items focused on access to care, satisfaction with hospital and medical care, utilization of services, and health outcomes (using twenty items from the Medical Outcomes Study). Bindman indicates that the effect of hospital closure may be to increase problems of access to care and functional health status one year after closure. This is the only study of which we are aware in which data are presently available on the immediate health effects among the population formerly served by a hospital that closed.

There are several limitations of the study, one of which is its focus on *patients* of the two hospitals, and not on the general population. This is precisely the problem addressed by Deuschle, who pointed out that it is not the *constituency* of a hospital, but the *health of the community* it serves that gives an indication of the impact of its closure (Deuschle, 1983). If we really want to understand the way in which a "community-focused" caregiving program is perceived, we must seek an answer among a population larger than those who actually *use* its services. The emphasis should be less on *rural hospitals* per se and more on the *health care of rural people*.

A fourth study of relevance to our present focus is an investigation of the determinants of consumer demand for collectively provided goods and services conducted by Fort and Christianson, which analyzed voting behavior on rural hospital referenda in ten states (Colorado, Idaho, Kansas, Montana, Nebraska, Nevada, North Dakota, South Dakota, Utah, and Wyoming) during the period from 1946 to 1978 (Fort and Christianson, 1981). Information provided through surveys of 542 county clerks in these states identified 152 health care referenda during this thirty-two-year period. Sixty-nine of these referenda had to do only with hospitals and were selected for analysis. The categories of explanatory variables (i.e., predictors of referenda success) selected for inclusion in the study were (1) the level of hospital capital that would prevail under passage of the referendum; (2) the level of capital associated with referendum failure; (3) the average income of the county population; (4) expected income changes owing to passage or failure of the referendum; (5) the prices of collectively provided hospital capital to the representative resident of the county; and (6) the value of intergovernmental grants. Unfortunately, proxy measures were introduced for most of the principal explanatory variables in the study. In addition, because it was anticipated that aggregate voting results would be influenced by the size of population groups likely to be high demanders of health care services, two variables were introduced into the analysis: the percentage of the county population over 65 years of age and the birth rate per thousand population in the county.

Many of the hypothesized relationships did not turn out to be that significant, but it was interesting to note that counties with higher concentrations of elderly did not seem to prefer present hospital capital investments through taxation, presumably because they did not see themselves as likely to benefit from these investments. Furthermore, the proposed increases in per capita expenditures for hospital care did not, in and of themselves, enhance the probability of referenda passage, all else remaining equal. Most of these hospital referenda tended to pass, despite rather high levels of dissatisfaction with levels of public expenditures for hospital services.

The most salient finding of this study for our present purposes is that support for rural hospitals and opposition to rural hospital closures will be strong in counties with relatively low personal property taxes and high concentrations of benefiting groups (e.g., groups with a high birth rate, or persons engaged in retail and wholesale trade, who are likely to be supporters of rural hospital referenda because they receive concentrated benefits from an increase in hospital capital). Those voters who are likely to gain the most from an increase in hospital capital expansion are more likely to vote than are other rural residents. These voters/beneficiaries are likely to argue that the utility gains from increasing public indebtedness to finance hospital capital expansion are preferable to the utility losses likely to be realized by aversion to increasing debt.

A Proposed Framework for the Study of Rural Hospital Consumer Behavior and Preferences

The literature we have reviewed here indicates the limited extent to which issues related to consumer choice have been studied in the field of rural health services research. Yet there are a number of fairly recent examples of studies that have tried both to conceptualize and to measure some of the more important dimensions of rural consumer preferences and shopping behavior related to hospital and physician services. The variables that have been most often identified in this rather narrow literature are of two general types: (1) variables that describe or index the characteristics of *hospitals,* and (2) variables that define properties of the health care *consumer behavior* of those who use these facilities and services. In table 10.1, we list the most

Table 10.1. Variables of Importance to the Study of
Hospital Services Use

Variables that index hospital characteristics	Variables related to consumer behavior and preferences	
Ownership status	Age, gender, race, education, income, occupation	Proportion of population 65 years of age
Occupancy rate	Insurance coverage	Proportion of population employed in wholesale or retail trade
Competitive beds within service area	Attitudes re hospital billing practices	Beliefs and attitudes re value of health
Scope of services offered by hospital	Attitudes re local physician services	Length of residence in the community
County population change in previous decade	Local physician as source of primary care	Pattern of use of physician in previous community of residence
Presence of skilled nursing or other long-term care unit in county	Distance to primary care physician	Personal mobility (vacations, work, transportation availability)
Joint Commission accreditation	Length of time in association with primary care physician (loyalty)	Health status (perceived and measured)
Membership in multiinstitutional system	Physician care in previous year	Attitudes toward quality of local services
Ability to provide high-technology care	Specialized health care needs	Attitudes toward (image of) local community
Length of stay	Mix of local medical specialties	Level of local personal property taxes
Average case-mix severity	Mix of local medical/health problems of consumer/patient	Estimated travel time to each of area health care facilities
	Perceived capacity and responsiveness of local hospital emergency room	Knowledge of, familiarity with, and attitudes toward local hospital
	Proportion of children in local population (birth rate/1000)	

important variables in each category. Future research in this area should seek to build upon these efforts.

Policy Options for Addressing the Rural Hospital Situation

The principal thrust of public policy considerations in relation to the future of the rural hospital in the United States appears to take one of two basic strategic approaches:

1. To move in the direction of restructuring *individual hospital facilities* so as to make them into facilities providing different (usually lower) levels of health care, meeting specific types of health needs in the communities they serve
2. Integrating groups of rural health care facilities (including general hospitals) into multiinstitutional *systems of care* wherein separate facilities agree to provide different levels of care through an arrangement that involves the systematic transfer of patients from one level of facility to another as the need arises.

Elements of both of these approaches were represented in the Omnibus Budget Reconciliation Act of 1989 passed by the 101st Congress. That legislation describes the so-called "Rural Primary Care Hospital" as a low-intensity, subacute, or limited care hospital meeting basic acute and primary care health needs. These facilities will be expected to provide emergency acute care services and have no more than six holding beds capable of meeting patient needs for up to seventy-two hours of care. Formal arrangements for patient transfer and referral to Essential Access Community Hospitals (EACHs), Rural Referral Centers, and urban hospitals must be worked out as part of the funding and certification process.

An EACH is a facility of no fewer than seventy-five beds (a requirement that can be waived) that is located no less than thirty-five miles or forty-five minutes from another EACH or a Rural Referral Center. Emphasis in the House legislation is on the development of rural consortia arrangements among a number of existing facilities in the process of application and their designation as "systems" of rural health care at the time federal funding is granted.

Each of these general strategies (one focused on transitions in the organization of and services offered by an individual hospital, the other focused on the formation of multiinstitutional health care consortia and systems of care) may be classified as strategies for *hospital conversion*. Two distinct forms of hospital conversion have been identified (Gibbens and Ludtke, 1989): (1) conversion *within a level of care* (i.e., the facility essentially reduces its level of service activity in order to provide a lower intensity of acute medical and hospital care); and (2) conversion *between levels of care* (i.e., the hospital undertakes to become a different type of facility, such as a provider of long-term or primary health care). Many states have already passed legislation to assist existing rural hospitals with such conversions, or to enable local communities to reinstate a formerly closed facility as another type of health care provider organization meeting a different type of need.

Although this brief overview of the principal thrust of recent Congressional legislative proposals for addressing the special problems of rural hospitals does not intend to describe thoroughly the detailed provisions of either state or federal initiatives, it does suggest certain aspects of current policy options that must be included in any national survey of rural consumer preferences. Among these are:

- The receptivity of rural residents to the receipt of emergency room, outpatient hospital care, and acute observational care in facilities from which they might have to be moved in the event that more advanced levels of care would be required
- The willingness of rural residents to travel as far as thirty-five miles (or forty-five minutes) in order to obtain full-service (secondary level) hospital care
- The willingness of rural residents to be cared for during the initial stages of hospitalization by nurse practitioners and/or physician's assistants, rather than by physicians, prior to transfer to a full-service hospital if that should be necessary
- The degree of support among rural residents for the conversion of existing hospital facilities in their communities to alternative levels of care (e.g., long-term care or primary care)

Defining the Service Areas of Focal Hospitals. It would be our suggestion that considerable effort go into defining the "reasonable geographic boundaries" of the service areas of rural hospitals.

This process should involve exploring the availability of local patient origin data and the determination of which telephone exchanges represent reasonable geographic boundaries of these areas.

Identifying Alternative Providers of Hospital Services. In each of these service areas (or in areas adjacent to them) effort should be made to plot the location, interfacility distance, and respective characteristics of alternative sources of hospital care. The characteristics of these hospital care options have been shown to have much to do with the way in which small rural hospitals are viewed and used.

The Structure and Content of Survey Instruments or Questionnaires. The survey instrument for the study of consumer choices in rural hospital care should include the following basic component segments of questions:

- *Basic sociodemographic information.* This should include age, race, gender, income, occupation, and education.
- *Residential history.* Here the focus should be on whether the individual ever lived elsewhere, whether there are strong ties with the community(ies) in which he or she may have lived before, and whether he or she may have established ties with health care providers in these communities.
- *Image of the local community, job, home.* It should be the objective to know more about the way in which the individual views the local community and his or her identification with it and its future.
- *Personal mobility.* It is important to gain a better understanding of travel patterns for vacations, work, and shopping, and the availability of personal means of transportation (e.g., a car, truck, or public transport), or the need to pay one's friends or neighbors for transportation to stores or for medical care. Here we are interested in obtaining an index of conventional patterns of mobility related to shopping for nonmedical goods and services that might take place out of the local community.
- *Distance to hospital and medical care.* A study of this kind should obtain the respondent's estimate of the distance and travel time from his or her residence to local hospitals (the focal hospital plus principal alternatives) and physician services normally used in time of need.

- *Hospital use in the previous year.* Information should be collected on the extent to which members of the household have used any kind of hospital service in the previous year and the name and location of the hospital.
- *Perceptions of the local hospital.* It is important to explore the respondent's knowledge of, familiarity with, attitudes toward, and image of the local hospital, and, wherever possible, comparable measures for the most important alternative sources of hospital care. The fundamental issue here is to what extent the respondent correctly understands the kind of care currently available in and through the local hospital. In addition, we should measure, much as was done by Ben-Sira (1983), the "image" of the local hospital, to include measures of perceptions of the hospital's level of professional competency, the quality of medical care given by the hospital's physicians, and the affective behavior of physicians and nurses, and overall satisfaction with care received in the past.
- *Loyalty to the local hospital.* A study of this kind will require estimates of both attitudinal and behavioral loyalty to the local hospital. We are attracted to the approach to the measurement of hospital loyalty recommended by MacStravic (1987). This approach draws on product marketing experience in other fields and includes questions asking the respondent to assign to the hospital a priority position in a list of possible sources of hospital care. For example:

> When you think of a hospital, what is the first one that comes to mind?
> 1 = the focal hospital
> 0 = none or noncompeting hospital
> –1 = competing hospital
> Why is that? _____

(MacStravic, 1987, 26–27)

This measure also includes items measuring the extent of use of any hospital and whether use occurred at the focal or some other hospital. In addition, questions are included measuring the preference of the respondent for which hospital they would like to go to if hospitalization were necessary. For example:

> If you were admitted to a hospital, which would be your personal choice?

1 = the focal hospital
0 = no preference
−1 = competing hospital
What makes that hospital your best choice? _____

Based on your personal physician's affiliation, where would you expect to be admitted if you needed to be admitted to a hospital?
1 = the focal hospital
0 = no preference
−1 = competing hospital

If you were scheduled for admission to (the focal hospital) but no beds were available, would you go to another hospital or wait for a bed in (other preferred hospital) assuming there was no danger in waiting?
2 if (preferred hospital) = focal hospital and would wait
1 if (preferred hospital) = focal hospital and would switch
−1 if (preferred hospital) = another hospital and would switch
−2 if (preferred hospital) = another hospital and would wait
Why is that? _____

- *About the respondent's personal physician.* Here it is important to know where the physician's office is located, how long the respondent has been associated with the physician, and the extent to which the respondent (and other members of the household) have used physician services in the previous year.
- *Personal health status.* It would be useful to obtain a measure of the personal health status of the respondent and other household members, to include measures of specialized care needs and the extent to which health-related disability has restricted functional status or other activities in the previous year. Such variables can have a substantial impact on health care utilization behavior and on the attitudes about the care received.
- *Response to illness symptoms and accidents.* Measures will be necessary of the likely response to given symptoms of illness, varying in degree of acuity and severity, and the places where members of the household would be likely to seek medical and hospital care in the event that a need arose.
- *Preferences with regard to hospital care availability.* Here it will be important to explore the distance (or time) respondents would be willing to travel in search of medical and hospital care. This would be the point at which we would pose the questions having to do with willingness to seek first-echelon medical and hospital care at a facility that was equipped to provide primary care and limited emergency and observational in-

patient services, with arrangements for transfer to other more sophisticated facilities in the event that these higher levels of care were needed.

With these sets of items, the proposed study should be able to characterize patterns of hospital and medical care use in ways not heretofore possible in other studies. Moreover, the specific and intended effect of policy options currently under review or enacted by law could be presented to respondents. Data from the study would permit the estimation of the extent to which residents of these communities would be accepting of these proposed arrangements, and would allow for the comparison of these hypothetical patterns of use with previous utilization of existing hospital and medical care facilities and services.

Summary

The literature on the stability and performance of the rural hospital in the United States is in need of a new direction and focus. We have acquired a clear picture of the structural and environmental characteristics of rural hospitals that have fallen into conditions of economic stagnation or have closed. We have even gained a perspective on the geographic patterns of use of these facilities by the communities they were intended to serve. What is missing is a more complete picture of the values (or utilities) that rural community residents place on having hospital services of different levels (e.g., inpatient acute and intensive care, outpatient medical and surgical care, long-term care, and emergency services) available in and through their local hospital. Moreover, we know far too little about the complex relationship between services available in a local hospital and patterns of use of local physician services. As new proposals are advanced for transforming the small rural hospital into a different kind of health care facility, such information will become even more important as the basis for sound social policy in this area. The field of health services research has much to contribute to the state of knowledge in the health services field and our understanding of the feasibility of new programs addressing these important social problems in rural America. The proposals we have made here would help to meet these needs.

Chapter 11

Emergency Medical Services in Rural Areas

ROBERT RUTLEDGE, THOMAS C. RICKETTS, AND ELIZABETH BELL

It has been estimated that the average American will need ambulance service at least twice in his or her lifetime, and, for some of these patients, delays in receiving emergency care may contribute to increased morbidity or mortality (Wears, 1989). The one-quarter of Americans who live in rural areas face unique problems in obtaining emergency care. Although the number of deaths that occur in rural areas are roughly equivalent in raw numbers to the number that occur in urban areas, the large land area covered, the widely dispersed populations, and the small rural communities present a difficult management problem. This chapter will describe the unique characteristics of emergency medical services (EMS) in the rural environment, focusing on the problems of trauma care and the structure of trauma services.

Emergency Medical Services and Rural America

During the past ten years, there have been major changes in the U.S. health care system. In rural areas, this change has been associated with a decline in local economies and the closing of many rural hospitals. Since 1981, nearly 550 rural hospitals have closed (Merlis, 1989). This trend is associated with the loss of hospital-based care and subsequent decrease in ready access to EMS.

Access to well-trained personnel, essential equipment, and facilities in rural communities that lack a local hospital or physician continues to be problematic (Anderson et al., 1986). Sometimes this access can be arranged through cooperation with neighboring communities that have such medical resources. As the availability of centralized hospital care and medical care decreases, EMS providers have had to assume new and increased responsibilities (Certo et al., 1983; Krob et al., 1984). There is often an increased demand for nonemergency transport to and from hospitals and to and from urgent primary care services.

Specific problems for rural EMS systems are the low population density in rural areas; poor roads, which can cause EMS transport delays; and difficulty in public access because of limited implementation of 911 systems throughout the states. Rural residents often must make long-distance telephone calls to obtain emergency assistance—and some rural areas continue to be without telephone service. In addition, communications via UHF and VHF frequencies are continually plagued by "dead spots" and crowded radio frequencies, which limit communications between rural emergency medical technicians (EMTs) and hospital-based physicians. There are limitations in the availability of prehospital care providers, the majority of whom are volunteers. Available rural prehospital care providers often have only basic levels of training (Donovan et al., 1989). Rural EMS providers have difficulty maintaining specialized skills to handle emergencies owing to the low volume of EMS calls and the low volume of emergencies within this total volume. There are limited numbers of rural physicians trained to provide appropriate medical supervision for EMS operations. Equipment is limited and aeromedical transport is available only in rare situations. Rural hospital emergency room physicians and nurses often do not have advanced EMS training (Larson and Mellstrom, 1987). EMS hospitals may not have EMS protocols, localized equipment may not be available, and trauma systems and their implementation may not be available. Rural areas often lack the resources (basically financial) needed to address EMS problems.

Rural trauma is a major problem in the United States. According to such studies as that by the National Academy of Sciences, up to 70 percent of trauma fatalities occur in rural areas, even though 70 percent of the population live in urban areas (Baker et al., 1987, 1988; National Academy of Sciences, 1966). Over the past three decades, numerous studies have defined the concept of preventable trauma death in both rural and urban populations. By its nature, rural trauma is difficult to study. Data sources have routinely focused on injuries occurring in urban areas. However, with the development of large data sources that include greater numbers of patients, samples are available with enough rural patients to draw conclusions about rural trauma. Data described in this chapter show that recommendations derived from urban trauma experience may not apply to rural patients.

Agriculture is considered the most dangerous occupation in the United States, and, unlike other occupations, children make up a significant portion of the workforce (National Coalition for Agricultural Safety and Health, 1988). Nearly 300 children and adolescents die each year from farm injuries, and approximately 23,500 suffer nonfatal trauma. The fatality rate increases with the age of the child. The rate for fifteen- to nineteen-year-old boys is double that of young children and 26 percent higher than that for girls. More than half (52.5 percent) die without ever reaching a physician; an additional 19.1 percent die in transit to a hospital, and only 7.4 percent live long enough to receive inpatient care. The most common cause of fatal and nonfatal injury is farm machinery. Tractors accounted for one-half of these machinery-related deaths, followed by farm wagons, combines, and forklifts. Overall, 10 percent of children with nonfatal injuries require hospitalization, and one in thirty children younger than the age of five years with a farm injury is hospitalized or dies. The magnitude of the problem requires the evaluation of a number of preventive strategies, including legislation and improvement of emergency care in rural areas.

The frequency of emergency events encountered by rural versus urban EMS systems has been evaluated. Cardiopulmonary resuscitation (CPR) is required in only a small percent of transports. Rural ambulance services are often staffed by volunteers. These volunteers usually work a full-time regular job in addition to their work staffing the EMS, therefore, most are capable of accepting staff coverage of the EMS on only a limited basis. Given the low frequency of CPR, it has been estimated that it may take five years for an individual member of a rural EMS team to be faced with a single episode of cardiopulmonary arrest. This means that rural volunteers' experience with emergency events, such as cardiopulmonary arrest, will be severely limited.

This limited exposure to emergency events has implications for EMS systems. Suggestions that rural emergency medical care can be improved by increasing the training provided to rural emergency medical providers must take this situation into account. Because of the large number of rural EMS providers, such training programs would be expensive. A large investment to improve EMT skills throughout rural areas might not be effective because of problems with skill retention. It would be very difficult for the rural providers to maintain their skill level in the management of emergency events when their experience is so limited. The fact that rural EMS and hospital staff may be called upon very infrequently to assess and stabilize patients with injuries as severe as those seen by their urban colleagues has major implications for rural trauma management and organization.

Yet even though EMS systems and system providers in rural areas may have difficulty in maintaining the specialized skills necessary for management of emergencies; well-organized EMS systems are essential components of medical care. For rural residents, for whom no local hospital or other medical care may be available, the EMS system may be particularly important in allowing residents to maintain their health.

History of Emergency Medical Services

EMS and emergency medicine in general are relatively new areas of health care (Sanders, 1989). As recently as twenty years ago, there was an absence of responsibility for EMS. Unlike police and fire services—with their high visibility and strong national organization, with a position of prominence at both state and local levels—ambulance services were often neglected and ignored. Many were run by funeral homes and most were staffed by inadequately trained individuals with minimal medical backgrounds. Hospital emergency departments were often understaffed, disorganized, and not committed to the emergency medical care of their surrounding communities (D. D. Boyd et al., 1983). In addition, little research was directed at illness management prior to hospitalization. But during the past two decades, there has been a remarkable change in emergency medical services in the United States. Over the past twenty-five years, the American College of Surgeons, the American Health Association, the National Safety Council, the American Academy of Orthopaedic Surgeons, the American Medical Association, the American

Hospital Association, and the Joint Commission on Accreditation of Health Care Organizations have established new standards for emergency medical technicians, and medical and nursing schools are now giving greater attention to emergency care. Emergency medicine has emerged as a distinct new specialty with appropriate scientific and organizational support.

Congressional concern about emergency medical services was initiated through the National Highway Safety Act in 1966. This act authorized the U.S. Department of Transportation (DOT) to set guidelines for EMS. The DOT provided funds for the purchase of ambulances and equipment, the installation of communication systems, the development of widespread support of EMT training programs and the development of the first statewide EMS plans. Also under this law, federal funds were allocated to each state on a block grant basis that are matched by state resources. Funds are distributed through each Governor's Highway Safety Representative on a largely unpublished basis for each of the sixteen approved Highway Safety Standards. The most widely known result of the DOT programs was the development of the emergency medical technician as a new health professional. This has become widely accepted as the minimal level of training required for persons treating patients at the emergency scene or en route to a hospital via ambulance. DOT continues to support training programs as well as the purchase of vehicles and equipment, though their total available EMS funds have decreased. DOT was also the initial supporter of the Military Assistance and Safety and Traffic Program, using military helicopters to assist in emergency transport prior to the advent of hospital-based helicopters. This was one of the early attempts at emergency transport over long distances, particularly in rural areas in North Carolina.

In 1972 the Health Services and Mental Health Administration was designated as the lead agency for EMS within what is now the Department of Health and Human Services (DHHS). A program to develop five "total EMS systems" was launched. The primary purpose was to develop and demonstrate various approaches to providing emergency medical care in a systematic and comprehensive manner so that other states and communities could gain from these experiences. The common thread in each of these projects was emphasis on a regional approach to emergency medical care. It became increasingly accepted that all hospitals could not provide comprehensive EMS systems and that our society could not afford unnecessary competition and duplication of effort. The emphasis on shared resources and a regional approach has been substantiated and continues today.

On November 4, 1973, P.L. 93-154 was enacted. Its purpose was to provide incentives for appropriate governmental units to inventory their resources for providing comprehensive EMS care, to identify gaps in such services, to remedy these deficiencies through better coordination and utilization of existing resources, and to develop the components essential to achieve an integrated comprehensive EMS system. The legislation sought to integrate the following elements into regional EMS systems: personnel, training, communications, transportation, facilities, critical care units, public safety agencies, consumer participation, accessibility to care, transfer of patients, standardized patient record-keeping, public information and education, independent review and evaluation, disaster linkage, and mutual aid agreement. The United States was divided into 300 EMS regions and over a quarter of the country received federal support under the law for developing basic life support regional EMS systems.

Trauma in Rural Areas

As noted previously, trauma death rates have been shown to be higher in rural than in urban counties (Rutledge et al., 1990; Spears, 1986). But rurality does not explain all the variation in per capita trauma death rates. For example, rural counties in eastern North Carolina have higher mortality rates than similarly rural counties in the western part of the state, suggesting that factors other than or in addition to rurality contribute to the increased mortality in these counties. Analysis of North Carolina data has demonstrated association of this higher mortality rate with differences in socioeconomic status, types of occupational and other exposures, and lower availability of prompt emergency care (Rutledge et al., 1990). Efforts to improve the quality of trauma care in rural communities include physician and nurse education, institution of trauma protocols promoting prompt resuscitation and stabilization of patients, regular trauma case reviews, and EMT and prehospital management coordination (Wayne, 1989).

Although the rates of pedestrian injuries are higher in urban areas, the pedestrian fatality rate in rural areas is higher for nearly all age groups, and at all posted speeds (Mueller et al., 1988). A larger proportion of fatalities occurred outside the hospital and within the first hour after injury in rural areas than in urban areas. This finding is consistent with the idea that EMS is less available and that accessibility to trauma centers is more limited in rural areas.

A retrospective study was done in five Washington and Idaho communities to determine the incidence of severe trauma seen in small rural hospitals (Smith et al., 1985). Of the cases reviewed, 3.4 percent of the cases had an injury severity score (ISS) greater than or equal to 20, reflecting severe multisystem trauma, and 14.7 percent had an ISS of 10–19, reflecting severe trauma limited to one body system or multisystem trauma of a less critical nature; 5.3 percent of the patients had critical head injuries, 4.2 percent had major chest injuries, and 3.7 percent had serious abdominal injuries. The results showed that each individual physician or hospital did not see the severe cases often, but that, when they occurred, these types of injuries necessitated an experienced, rapid response on the part of the hospital staff. This finding has significant implications for trauma management in rural communities.

Case fatality studies provide important information on trauma care, but cannot assess adequately the full spectrum of serious injuries seen by rural hospital and prehospital personnel. A retrospective study was performed by Smith (1987) to examine the incidence of severe trauma seen in a small rural hospital. The results show once again that the incidence of severe trauma is not high, but that, when it occurs, these patients have injuries requiring aggressive early management for optimal outcome.

Cales and Trunkey (1985) have shown that trauma deaths have a trimodal distribution: approximately 50 percent of deaths occur within seconds to minutes of the accident, 30 percent occur within the first two to three hours, and 20 percent occur after days to weeks of hospitalization, usually from secondary medical complications. Thirty percent in the middle group are the persons that will benefit from acute medical interventions. Thus the period between two and three hours after the accident is called the "golden hour" of trauma care. Patient assessment, stabilization, and transport will continue to be the key parts of the golden hour of care. Regionalization of rural trauma care, with the development of tertiary referral centers and rapid air transport, has definitely contributed to improved patient outcomes. However, bypassing community hospitals and transporting patients directly to a larger center will not in and of itself improve patient survival. Regional centers and transport services must be used appropriately. They are not substitutes for accurate initial patient assessment, airway management, fluid replacement, and similar measures. In rural areas, these initial resuscitation decisions and actions will usually still be made and implemented by prehospital and emergency room personnel with physician backup as soon as available. Rural hospital and EMS personnel must be prepared to deal with clinically ill patients with major traumatic injuries: these patients require aggressive early treatment if morbidity and mortality are to be reduced, and, despite advances in air transport and regionalization of prehospital care, rapid access to tertiary trauma centers will continue to be difficult logistically for many trauma victims in rural areas such as those described in Smith's study. The challenge facing those in leadership positions is how to provide a rural health care delivery system to meet these needs. Medical and paramedical personnel in rural communities must have the skills available to stabilize and appropriately refer patients with severe trauma. Regional backup services for both acute referrals and continuing education are essential.

Waller (1974; Waller et al., 1966) noted that urban-oriented methods fail to solve rural emergency care problems. He went on to identify a number of problems that are unique to rural areas: the limited number of physicians in hospitals in rural communities, a shortage of persons with trauma management skills and experience, low population density with consequently long distances and poor roads, and limited financial resources. Not surprisingly, more than fifteen years later, these continue to be major problems facing rural trauma care. Waller also documents how infrequently ambulance crews are called upon to handle severe emergencies and suggests that this lack of experience contributes to their difficulty in maintaining adequate clinical skills.

Components of Emergency Medical Services Systems

The handling of emergency cases depends on close coordination of multiple community resources in an organized system (American College of Emergency Physicians, 1988a,b; 1987; American

College of Surgeons, 1986, 1987). Past neglect is now being over-come, but many communities still rely on a fragmented and inad-equate system of transportation, communication, and hospital and physician services. Hospitals have frequently been concerned primarily with their own needs to the exclusion of community needs. Ambulance, police, and fire departments have also contrib-uted to some conflict in directions for emergency care.

EMS systems include the personnel, vehicles, equipment, and facilities used to deliver medical care to those outside of the hospi-tal setting. The primary goals of EMS systems are to provide immediate medical assistance at the scene and while in transit to medical care facilities, to provide rapid transportation to a medi-cal support facility, and to have a coordinated system of hospitals so that the most seriously ill individuals can be quickly taken to specialized care facilities and the less severely ill or injured pa-tients cared for locally. Comprehensive EMS *systems* have been shown to save lives and reduce morbidity and mortality from illness and injury (Ornoto et al., 1985; Urdaneta et al., 1987). Among the EMS system components that are required are rapid public access, on-the-scene emergency care personnel, rapid trans-port, physician-trained EMS supervision, levels of hospital care for appropriate management, and EMS surveillance systems to facilitate continued quality assurance and appropriate resource utilization in the system.

Identifying the need for and effecting appropriate changes in the system must be based upon a complete and accurate descrip-tion of illness events and EMS and medical system responses. Evaluation of EMS care is difficult. Most of the care occurs in a noncentralized location, there is much disagreement about appro-priate management techniques, and little information is available on outcomes of EMS intervention. Adequate outcome measures, other than life and death, have been difficult to obtain. Outcome assessment during the patient's course from onset of the illness or injury through hospitalization, discharge, and rehabilitation is needed for proper evaluation of the EMS system.

Consideration of the financial aspects of out-of-hospital EMS is essential to an understanding of the problems and opportunities facing regional EMS systems. The availability of financial support from both public and private sources has stimulated widespread interest and considerable progress in development of regional EMS systems, but not many communities have adequately addressed the cost and revenue implications of EMS systems. Those seeking to make improvements and changes in an EMS system are always faced with the question of determining the cost of and securing the necessary financing for those changes. EMS system costs are related mainly to transportation, communications, and overall management. Transportation costs are based on personnel expense, administrative expense, medical supplies, vehicle operating and maintenance expense, garage and office expense, and vehicle equipment depreciation. Communications costs include dispatcher and crew expense, equipment maintenance, telephone service, and equipment depreciation. System management includes personnel expense, office expense, travel expense, and consultant services. The costs of EMS are influenced by multiple factors and vary from community to community. System structure, size, and sophistication as well as community characteristics all affect cost. Studies of overall EMS operating costs, including hospital costs, indicate that they range from $7 to $15 per person in the area served (Health Economics Research, 1988). Out of this total, between $2 and $4 covers out-of-hospital services. DHHS estimates that EMS costs range between $4 and $7.50 per resident based on whether basic or advanced life support training has been provided to personnel.

Costs and Financing of Rural Emergency Medical Services

The cost of operating an ambulance service typically ranges between 20 and 30 percent of total EMS system cost. Personnel cost, the largest portion of ambulance service costs, is often as high as 60–90 percent. Training costs are based largely upon the type and sophistication of the training provided. The burden of these and other fixed costs—those incurred regardless of the number of runs made and thus likely to have the greatest impact in situations of underutilization—is most apparent in EMS transportation services in rural regions. Substantial fixed costs result in the high cost of maintaining adequate ambulance response capability in sparsely populated areas, and therefore per capita costs generally reflect a strong inverse relationship to population density; that is, per capita costs increase as distance traveled increases and as the number of runs decreases. Rural populations are then faced with particular problems in maintaining adequate EMS systems.

Communications costs associated with EMS may range from as little as 2 percent of the total where costs are shared with other public services to as much as 35 percent in rural areas where extensive communication networks are maintained solely for EMS purposes. Again, the rural situation presents a difficult problem for appropriate management. System management costs are also widely variable, depending on the local arrangements.

There are usually two different types of funding sources. One is initial developmental or grant funds that are made available by the federal government (principally the DOT and the DHHS), state governments, and private foundations. The second principal source is operational funding, which is directed toward the ongoing expenses of the system. The availability of funds to meet developmental expenses led to the startup of EMS systems around the country. In many cases, however, there have been major problems in maintaining permanent financing for ongoing systems. Service charges and subscriptions are major sources of operating funds for emergency transportation. Ambulance services typically charge a base fee with additional mileage charges and supplementary charges for special services. Charges vary but tend to be higher in urban than in rural areas. In urban areas, a fixed fee is quite common. With rural ambulance services, a mileage charge is routinely added.

Collection rates are poor for most ambulance services, ranging between 30 and 50 percent of charges. However, some groups have achieved collection rates of up to 80 percent through persistent pursuit of delinquent accounts. In many areas, local governments subsidize a portion of ambulance operating costs. The means for determining the method of subsidy and the amount of the subsidy vary. As a rule, the costs of EMS communications and system management are borne by local taxpayers or by developmental funds, where grant support is available.

EMS financing remains disorganized and fragmented. From a financial standpoint, EMS is still operating not as a system, but rather as a collection of unrelated elements. This is especially evident when current third-party financing provisions are considered. On the average, 80 percent of EMS patients are covered under one or more health insurance plans, such as Blue Cross, Blue Shield, Medicare, Medicaid, commercial insurance, and private programs. Those in rural areas are twice as likely to be covered as those in urban areas. At present, though, many insurance policies do not provide coverage for out-of-hospital emergency medical services, and policies that do include out-of-hospital benefits typically limit the nature and extent of coverage. Few health insurance plans specify any coverage for either communications or system management costs where they are not included in the transportation charges. In addition, common insurance restrictions often limit coverage to selected patient conditions, set maximum allowable costs for services, and/or restrict benefits to hospital-based services. Some commercial policies provide benefits for EMS transportation services only for patients hospitalized following transportation. Therefore, benefits have not kept pace with EMS financing needs.

Getting EMS systems to the public is a largely economic issue. In general, it takes between $200,000 and $300,000 to maintain a twenty-four-hour advanced life support (ALS) vehicle 365 days a year. An EMS system is a public service and the public must pay for the service, whether it is a purely tax-supported system, a purely private-provider system supported by direct billing of the patient, or some combination of systems. The development of an EMS system and the funding of it require careful planning and an accurate assessment of needs. Per capita expenditures for EMS systems in 1988 ranged from a low of $.02 in Ohio to nearly $14.00 in Hawaii (Office of Technology Assessment, U.S. Congress, 1989). Calculations of cost-benefit ratios have been proposed by a number of authors, using numbers of lives saved after cardiac arrest as a model. These estimates of cost per life saved are extremely variable, ranging from $4,300 per life saved by establishing a basic life support (BLS) ambulance alone to $42,358 per life saved after the establishment of an ALS system. The methodology for calculation of these numbers is so variable and complex that it is often obscure. As we have seen, personnel expenses total 60–90 percent of the costs of a typical system. Because of the high cost of personnel, many municipalities have used their fire departments as EMS providers. This makes more efficient use of a resource that is traditionally underutilized and is already designed to respond quickly to emergency calls. In rural areas, EMS systems have often been staffed by volunteers.

The costs of equipment are also significant in the development and operational stages. The cost of purchasing and equipping a BLS ambulance is estimated at $35,000 to $40,000. The cost of an ALS unit is approximately $80,000. The number of units required for a given area is dependent on population density, response time requirements, geographic area to be covered, and other demands for ambulance services. Generally accepted estimates for volumes of emergencies indicate that only 5 percent of all calls will be true emergencies and another 15 percent will require urgent evaluation, while the remainder will be nonemergency. An average of one medical emergency per day will be generated per 10,000 people. Because the fixed costs of EMS systems are so high, rural and wilderness systems that operate at low levels of efficiency are extremely expensive on a per capita basis.

In the 1980s, EMS services increasingly became a state responsibility. In 1980, over 80 percent of EMS funds were derived from state or local sources. A few states have directed the care of the seriously injured to designated trauma centers, but the majority do not designate specialized centers and lack regionalized systems of trauma care. Although a few states have developed model EMS systems that integrate rural and urban services, most have isolated, poorly organized rural EMS systems with limited resources.

Federal funding of state EMS activities is limited to support through the block grant program administered by the DHHS and through the DOT's National Highway Traffic Safety Administration. In 1988, $13 million of the DHHS block grant funds was spent by states on EMS while DOT distributed $5 million for EMS through the state and community Highway Safety Grant Program, Section 402. In recent years, EMS expenditures have declined sharply. Following the enactment of the 1973 EMS Systems Act, about $30 million was spent annually on EMS. In the early 1970s, as noted earlier, EMS systems were underequipped, poorly staffed, and fragmented. The goal of the EMS Act, to blanket the country with high-quality EMS programs, was not met before its demise in 1981, when the categorical programs, including EMS, were folded into the block grant program. This change led to a decline in EMS spending that has kept it well below 1970 levels. With new evidence of EMS fragmentation and inadequate resources, funding initiatives at the federal level are being improved, but are still limited.

Emergency Medical Services and Trauma Centers

An essential feature of the trauma center concept is the rapid delivery of patients with complicated injuries to a regional trauma center directly from the site of injury. Trauma patients treated at non–trauma center hospitals have worse outcomes than similarly injured patients treated at trauma centers (Houtchens, 1977). The proportion of preventable mortality is higher at non–trauma center hospitals, and the average costs and length of stay are increased in selected types of trauma treated in such hospitals. A variety of triage instruments have been proposed to aid prehospital personnel in making this difficult decision (Hawkins, 1988; Champion et al., 1981, 1991). The trauma score is a good predictor of early and late outcome for injured patients as well as a good predictor of the need for invasive procedures and for intensive care. This ability to predict outcome after injury rapidly and accurately can be used to decrease the mortality seen in patients injured in rural areas.

The goal in the care of the severely injured patient—treatment at a dedicated trauma center with as short a time interval as possible between the occurrence of trauma and the arrival of the patient at the trauma center—is often difficult to achieve, especially in rural areas of the country. The increased time required to get patients from rural areas to facilities that provide definitive trauma care may be a contributing factor to the higher rural trauma mortality rate (Garrison et al., 1989). In many rural areas, trauma patients are transported by ground prehospital EMS providers to the nearest community hospital, where an emergency physician must not only stabilize the patient but also arrange for transport to a trauma center. Whether emergency physicians in rural hospitals use available emergency helicopter services in a timely fashion and therefore take advantage of a resource that minimizes the time required to deliver definitive care to the trauma patient has not been assessed. There is no established standard or rule for how soon a referring physician should request a helicopter to transport a trauma patient under his or her care to a trauma center. Studies have demonstrated that the sooner a trauma victim arrives at a trauma center, the lower the probability of mortality and morbidity, especially if the patient gets to the trauma center within the so-called golden hour. Garrison's study demonstrates that there was often a lengthy period between the time of arrival of the trauma victim at the emergency department in rural eastern North Carolina and the time the trauma center was notified that helicopter service was needed. No objective factor could be correlated with the length of the interval. Patients who had predictably worse outcomes, as indicated by trauma score, ISS, the need for invasive intervention at the trauma center, and short-term mortality, were not transported sooner. Type of trauma, arrival time, day at the referral hospital, and distance of the referring hospital from the trauma center did not prompt earlier calls for the trauma helicopter service.

Prehospital trauma triage should permit accurate identification and transport of patients with critical injuries to trauma centers without overloading these centers with patients having minor injuries. In most trauma scoring systems, there is a combination of physiological criteria. Prehospital patient management decisions are complex because the traumatized patient population is heterogeneous with respect to demographics, mechanism of injury, physiological response to injury, and time from injury to medical care (Hedges et al., 1987). Hedges et al. (1987) found that on-scene time correlated linearly with a prolonged transport time. Hemodynamic and respiratory dysfunction was also associated with increased on-scene time. Mean on-scene time was not significantly different between high- and low-trauma-score groups, although patients with low trauma scores did receive more interventions (more intravenous lines, more frequent intubation, and more frequent pneumatic antishock garment use). The correlation of emergency department trauma score with initial prehospital trauma score and on-scene time demonstrated a small improvement in trauma score with increasing on-scene time for the patient with an initial trauma score greater than or equal to 13. However, patient groups with either low trauma scores or low Glasgow Coma Scores showed no significant improvement in trauma score with increasing on-scene time. Effective field triage of trauma victims requires identification of patients at risk of dying and their rapid transport to hospitals capable of treating severe injuries. Identification of these patients at the accident scene can be difficult, since prehospital personnel receive little training in structured triage decision-making.

The role of the physician in routine triage is disputed and his or her value has not been documented. Cottington et al. (1988) examined the influence of physiological, injury site, and injury mechanism criteria on the diagnosis of major trauma in 2,057 trauma patients because the trauma score was found to be a highly specific indicator of major trauma. Champion and Sacco (Landau et al., 1982; Champion et al., 1980, 1981) explored the severity of injury of three groups of trauma patients triaged by different guidelines to a Level 1 urban trauma center. Results showed that, with physician input in the triage process, patients chosen for helicopter transport to the trauma center had a significantly higher median level of injury severity than patients triaged to the trauma center without physician involvement. It has been suggested that, if triage criteria are to identify accurately patients with major trauma, not only physiological status but also anatomical site and injury mechanism must be assessed.

In recent years, trauma delivery has come under close scrutiny from within and outside the medical profession. With the development and designation of trauma centers, two problems have become evident. First is the need for a reliable, simple means of triaging patients to the appropriate facility. The second problem is evaluation of the quality of care provided. The assessment of results is difficult owing to the large number of variables (such as mechanisms of injury, anatomical sites of injury, and comorbidity) found in these patients and has led to the use of complex statistical analysis. The trauma score, originally developed as a triage tool, has also proven to be a reliable simple means of assessing the quality of care. The expected survival for each trauma score value has been established and each hospital's or surgeon's results can therefore be evaluated against that standard. A deviation from the expected survival curve may or may not be clinically significant as determined by a careful review of the patient's chart. The trauma score can be used as a quality assurance tool by any hospital or physician providing trauma services (Hawkins, 1988).

Helicopters and Rural Emergency Medical Service Systems

Aeromedical transport has evolved dramatically during the last forty-five years, again following the military-to-civilian path. It represents a real alternative to ground transport for rural emergency cases, and helicopter or fixed-wing systems are in use in every state except Maine and Hawaii (Missouri Health Facilities Review Committee, 1989). Aeromedical evacuation was utilized in a limited fashion during the closing years of World War II. During the Korean War, helicopter transport of the wounded became commonplace. The patient could only be carried outside the helicopter's cabin, however, so no medical care was rendered en route. In Vietnam, the patient was carried inside the helicopter and treatment was initiated during the flight. The concept of aeromedical transport was initiated in the civilian sector in 1972 in Denver, Colorado. Since then, over 100 medical helicopter programs have been implemented throughout the United States. Rapid transport is not the only service provided by the helicopter. Many of the sophisticated emergency medical procedures and interventions previously performed only in the hospital can now be brought to the patient and accomplished at the scene of the accident or during flight.

The use of helicopter transport and regionalization of trauma care have been suggested as means to improve the outcome of injured patients in rural areas. The rationale for the large expenditure to equip and staff helicopter programs has been to decrease the time interval from injury until definitive care is begun. The assumption has been that helicopter transport will significantly improve outcome by shortening transport time. However, as discussed earlier, studies have suggested that delays in calling for transport may be preventing the large investment in helicopter transport from improving outcome (Garrison et al., 1989). The time from injury until arrival at the trauma center is longer in patients who are initially triaged to another hospital. Delays of up to several hours in contacting the helicopter for transport have been reported. These delays then mitigate the potential effectiveness of helicopter utilization.

Comparison of Trauma Patient Outcome in Trauma Center and Non–Trauma Center Hospitals

The key study in comparing outcomes of trauma patients treated in trauma center and non–trauma center hospitals was that by Trunkey's group in Orange County, California (Cales, 1984; Cales and Trunkey, 1985). That study clearly demonstrated that the frequency of preventable death in trauma patients was higher in patients treated at non–trauma center hospitals. Despite this study, organized statewide approaches to the triage and care of trauma patients are rare. Further studies are needed to convince local government administrators, EMS directors, physicians, and hospital administrators that such transfer protocols are appropriate. In addition, even though the findings of the Orange County study are strong, their applicability to rural areas remains unconfirmed. Patients who are transferred to trauma centers from local hospitals have a higher mortality rate than patients who come directly from the scene of injury to the trauma center. An increased length of time from injury to arrival at a trauma center is associated with increased mortality.

The appropriate level of care for the rural sick or injured patient varies depending upon the nature and the severity of the illness. Here again, information on the care of the trauma patient can serve as a model for systematic approaches to EMS care in rural areas in general. The requirements for the appropriate care of the seriously injured trauma patient can be determined from analysis of interventions required to treat the injured patient. Trauma patients frequently arrive after regular working hours. The peak arrival time is 8:00 P.M. Trauma patients are admitted more frequently on Fridays, Saturdays, and Sundays—not normal working days for most hospitals. Up to 25 percent of all trauma patients require a computed tomography (CT) scan of the head. To care appropriately for those who need head CT scans thus requires CT scan availability twenty-four hours a day. Even large hospitals have had difficulty in maintaining twenty-four-hour immediate CT scan availability. In addition, 50 percent of injured patients are transferred immediately from the emergency department to either the operating room or the intensive care unit. Again, given the most likely arrival days and times for trauma patients, both the operating room and the intensive care unit must be available on a twenty-four-hour basis. The intensive care unit and the operating room require a variety of support staff and services. This in turn means that respiratory therapy, the blood bank, and laboratory support must be available twenty-four hours a day. These requirements together constitute huge expense, and trauma center readiness, with its multiple requirements, has been estimated to cost a hospital from $1 to $4 million a year.

What can be done to decrease delays occurring at the outside hospital? A triage system to bypass the local hospital has been recommended, but one of the important concerns of hospitals is that, by allowing triage of such patients, bypassing the hospital might become routine. The hospital might then expect to lose patient referrals, leading to a decrease in reimbursement and a worsening financial position. This is particularly important for small rural hospitals because of their difficult financial situation. Triaging patients to the trauma center and bypassing the local hospital has been viewed as an assault on their patient referral pool.

What is needed is a means of successfully addressing both these issues: the fear of rural hospitals that triage of injured patients to the trauma center will lead to a worsening financial picture, and the potential for delays at outside hospitals while the patient undergoes further evaluation.

The vast majority of trauma patients are not severely injured. Use of two different measures of severity of injury, the trauma score and the ISS, demonstrates that *80 percent* of patients have relatively high (nonsevere) trauma scores (ranging from 14 through 16), and relatively low injury severity scores (ranging from 1 through 10) (Champion et al., 1991). The injuries of these patients are relatively mild, and their mortality rate is extremely low. Because of this low risk of morbidity and mortality, these patients could be adequately cared for at a smaller hospital.

Trauma score has been shown to be a good predictor of outcome. Patients with low trauma scores frequently die and those with high trauma scores rarely die. The data demonstrate that those patients with low trauma scores are also likely to have higher incidences of complications, a greater need for immediate surgery, a longer length of stay in the intensive care unit, a need for more days on the ventilator, and a longer length of stay in the hospital.

Patients who are more severely injured are at significant risk of dying or of suffering a major complication. They pose a problem for the small rural hospital for a number of reasons. The more severely injured patient costs two to three times more to treat. Furthermore, studies have clearly demonstrated that reimbursement for trauma care is very poor, and it is worst for the most severely injured (U.S. General Accounting Office, 1991; Champion and Mabee, 1990). This is particularly problematic for the small rural hospital that is trying to control its financial situation. Thus, given that the severely injured make up a small minority of all injured patients, in contrast to what many small hospitals think, appropriate triage of the severely injured may actually be beneficial to the financial status of the small hospital as well as to patient care. It is therefore in the best interests of both the small, rural hospital and the patient to identify seriously injured trauma patients and to initiate early transfer of such patients to a trauma center.

The practice of patient evaluation frequently utilizes a variety of studies as well as surgeons, neurosurgeons, or other physician specialists. Yet the trauma score, an easily obtainable set of vital signs, and a superficial physical examination can be used to identify those patients who are severely injured and are likely to die or suffer major complications. Because it is relatively easy to obtain and requires no special equipment beyond a blood pressure cuff, the trauma score can be calculated in the field or in the emergency department by a nurse or EMT, and physician input is not mandatory. By using the trauma score, one can identify at an early point those patients who need more specialized care because of their increased risk of morbidity and mortality.

Standards for resuscitation and transfer of trauma patients have been defined by the American College of Surgeons Committee on Trauma. In a prospective study by Hicks, major departures from accepted standards of early care were found in the handling of more than 70 percent of trauma patients transferred to a regional trauma center (Leicht et al., 1986). As noted earlier, 70 percent of fatal accidents in the United States occur in rural regions (National Academy of Sciences, 1966). Studies concluded that the lower survival rate for the victims of rural accidents correlated well with the deficiencies in transportation to a source of definitive medical care and the lack of trained personnel, appropriate equipment, and adequate local medical facilities (Urdaneta et al., 1987).

Data from North Carolina, Texas, South Carolina, and New York agree in demonstrating differences in the EMS requirements of rural and urban residents (Spears, 1986). Transports from rural areas are more commonly for cardiac or central nervous system complaints compared to an increased likelihood of transport for injuries of the trunk, spine, and brain; lacerations; and penetrating trauma in urban areas. This finding may be related to the higher percentage of the elderly present in rural areas. In data from the Texas EMS system, confirmed by results from North Carolina, the majority of transports from rural areas were of patients age sixty-five or older. In urban areas, only roughly one-third of transports were of those older than sixty-five years.

The type of ambulance call can be graded as emergent, critical, or routine. It is notable that only a small percent of EMS transports in either rural or urban areas are emergent or critical. The vast majority are classed as urgent or routine. Injuries in rural areas are associated with a higher per capita death rate. Houtchens (1977) points out that the fatality rate for rural victims of auto accidents is 40 to 60 percent higher than that for urban victims with comparable injuries. In California, the trauma mortality per 100,000 population was reported as forty-six deaths for rural counties and seventeen for urban counties, a difference of almost 3 : 1. This is confirmed by data from North Carolina as well as other states. The excess mortality is present in injuries from motor vehicle accidents as well as other causes, except for falls. The etiology of the increased death rate from motor vehicle accidents is related to a variety of factors other than larger distances and differences in emergency medical care for crash victims, including lower access to trauma centers and definitive care. Other problems that could be related to increased mortality in rural areas include poor road conditions, travel at higher rates of speed, the use of utility vehicles that have less safety equipment, and decreased use of seat belts (which has been documented in North Carolina as well as in other states).

Certain factors in rural trauma, such as the large geographic areas that EMS systems must cover, will always present challenges to the health care delivery system. Another factor unique to rural trauma is the infrequent nature with which severe trauma cases are seen. North Carolina data confirm other studies that show that the frequency of EMS transports is much less in rural areas: the mean number of transports for rural EMS systems is approximately fifty-nine per month, compared to a mean of 257 transports per month for urban EMS systems. The types of EMS transports are also important: emergencies make up only 12 percent of EMS transports in rural North Carolina; the rest are nonemergency interhospital transfers and trips home from the hospital. This information demonstrates that, of the limited number of EMS transports that occur each month in rural areas, most are nonemergency. Such transports would not assist the EMT in maintaining his or her skill level in the management of critically ill patients.

Training for Rural Emergency Medical Services

Determining the level of training for personnel in rural EMS settings may be difficult. As noted previously, skills retention by rural volunteers who do not participate in life-threatening situations frequently is a real problem. In most rural areas, an EMS system cannot be developed to an acceptable level without volunteers. Most volunteers have a deep commitment to public service. However, they may not be adequately prepared to deal with the stresses that they encounter. They may pay their own way for training and supplies. They may also need additional support when involved in rescue operations involving friends or family members.

Medical control in a rural EMS system is complicated by time, distance, and sometimes inadequate communications. Training should be directed at teaching EMTs how to care for their patients over extended periods of time. Rural systems often require extensive use of indirect medical control, such as standing orders and protocols, for, in many rural systems, the hospital is unable to have a physician available 24 hours a day.

Options for the Future

Options to try to improve EMS care in rural areas include increasing the funding to provide assistance for improving the level of skills of rural prehospital and hospital-based EMS providers. This funding would include support of EMS training and continuing education and state recruitment and placement programs. Another option would be a reevaluation of the criteria for prehospital EMS providers, to review some of the standard prehospital interventions that are presently in use to determine whether or not these (e.g., the use of mast trousers) do indeed save lives or whether other interventions (e.g., the use of hypertonic saline) might be more valuable.

The next option would be development of national guidelines and standards for prehospital EMS providers. Nationwide standards could be developed for EMS facilities such as trauma centers that would delineate the appropriate roles of rural hospitals in a national trauma EMS care system. This would allow triage of patients to appropriate levels of care based on severity of injury or illness. Funding of technical assistance to state EMS offices could be increased, to develop communication systems, enhance management skills and billing procedures, promote public education, improve the delivery of aeromedical services to rural areas, develop statewide regional EMS surveillance systems and reporting practices, and implement and adhere to quality assurance programs. Other options would be to fund further EMS research and demonstration programs to encourage investigation of EMS-specific problems unique to rural areas and rural EMS providers, and to augment support for state and community highway safety grant programs and earmark funds from these grants for EMS systems. Finally, a new area of categorical grants for EMS could be developed with specific attention to rural areas. Allocation of federal resources could be tied to a demand for state plans for overall implementation of EMS systems.

Chapter 12

Geographic Variation and Health Expenditures

GREGORY R. NYCZ AND

JOHN R. SCHMELZER

It has been estimated that total annual per capita expenditures for health care in the United States will grow from approximately $2,500 in 1990 to over $5,500 in the year 2000. Such spending levels could consume over $1.5 trillion and comprise 15 percent of the gross national product (GNP) at the turn of the century. Government expenditures are projected to grow from $269 billion in 1990 to nearly $650 billion by the year 2000 (Division of National Cost Estimates, Office of the Actuary, Health Care Financing Administration, 1987). If realized, the growth in health expenditures is likely to fuel additional cost-containment efforts on the part of government and private payers, and intensify debate over the relationship between expenditures for medical care and the overall health of the population. The distribution of federal health care funds will continue to be influenced by federal cost-containment legislation. However, the performance of national payment schemes, designed to reimburse based on efficient production of services, may not be responsive to diverse local market circumstances and should be periodically evaluated for unintended adverse consequences.

This chapter provides background data on health expenditures and outlines the relative importance to rural areas of major funding sources and financing mechanisms for health care. It includes a discussion of recent federal cost-containment legislation that is presented in the context of its implications for rural health care delivery systems. Data are presented that summarize the geographic distribution of federal Medicare expenditures from a resource allocation perspective. The chapter concludes with a discussion of factors that influence variability of per capita expenditures and some suggestions for additional policy-relevant research.

Background

Health care expenditures grew at an average annual rate of more than 11 percent throughout the 1970s. During this period, health expenditures as a percent of the GNP expanded from 7.4 percent in 1970 to 9.1 percent in 1980. Although average annual growth dropped below double-digit levels in the 1980s, the share of GNP devoted to health expenditures continued to rise as increases in health expenditures outpaced growth in the general economy. By 1990 health expenditures were estimated to represent 12 percent of GNP (Division of National Cost Estimates, Office of the Actuary, Health Care Financing Administration, 1987). The relentless growth in health expenditures stimulated public and private cost-containment efforts, contributed to the growth of the nation's uninsured population, and shifted the focus of access issues away from traditional rural concerns related to the availability of medical resources to financial problems associated with the ability to pay for care. In a special report on access to health care, the Robert Wood Johnson Foundation concluded that the nation experienced a deterioration in access to medical care in the mid-1980s despite an expansion in medical providers, noting that "For almost 19 million Americans, the problem is financial (Robert Wood Johnson Foundation, 1987)."

The focus on expenditures and payment systems in a new "competitive" environment also influenced rural health advocates and some members of Congress. This influence was reflected in broadened rural health agendas that placed significant emphasis on concerns related to hospital and physician payment levels in rural areas. Examples of the growing importance of payment issues in the rural agenda include the following:

1. Specific recommendations for research related to payments to rural hospitals, rural alternative delivery systems, and rural primary care providers were incorporated as part of the rural research agenda developed in response to a Congressional directive (Hersh and Van Hook, 1989).

2. The House Rural Health Care Coalition and the National Rural Health Association incorporated Medicare reimbursement equity as major goals in 1989 (National Rural Health Association, 1989).
3. The NRHA filed a lawsuit against the Secretary of the Department of Health and Human Services challenging the constitutionality of the methodology used to determine Medicare reimbursement to rural hospitals (National Rural Health Association, 1988a).

Sources of Payment

Information on the distribution of health care costs by source of payment is helpful to understand better the relative importance of different payers in nonmetropolitan and metropolitan areas (see chapter 2 for definitions). A recent examination of major funding sources for health care indicates that in 1989 40.6 percent of total personal health care expenditures came from government sources, 35.9 percent from private third parties, and 23.5 percent from direct patient payments (Lazenby and Letsch, 1990). This major federal role in financing personal health care is primarily due to the Medicare program, which accounted for 46 percent of total government health expenditures in 1989 and is projected to account for nearly 56 percent in the year 2000. Because the elderly consume a disproportionate amount of hospital and physician services, Medicare is the largest single purchaser of hospital care and physician services in the nation, accounting for 26.7 percent of all hospital revenue and for 23.4 percent of physician services in 1989 (Lazenby and Letsch, 1990). Medicare's role as primary payer for nonmetropolitan delivery systems is even more pronounced given that the elderly comprise a larger proportion of the population in these areas (12.3 percent) than in metropolitan areas (10.4 percent) (Norton and McManus, 1989).

"Although one-quarter of all Americans live in rural areas, public funding for health care in rural America has consistently lagged behind the U.S. average. At the federal level, per capita expenditures for health and related services are far lower for rural residents: 42 percent fewer health service dollars per capita than the U.S. average, 50 percent fewer social service dollars per capita than the U.S. average" (National Association of Community

Health Centers and National Rural Health Association, 1988). Analysis of the National Medical Care Utilization and Expenditures Survey provides some added insight into metropolitan/nonmetropolitan differences in the form of average charges experienced by individuals for health care. Results indicate generally lower average total charges per capita for nonmetropolitan residents. However, nonmetropolitan residents appear to pay a higher portion of their total charges on an out-of-pocket basis (U.S. Health Care Financing Administration, 1985). The higher proportion of out-of-pocket expenditures by nonmetropolitan residents may be due in part to higher rates of rural uninsured (Dicker and Sunshine, 1988) and/or less comprehensive benefits for those with insurance (National Rural Electric Cooperative Association, 1988a,b).

Alternative Methods of Financing

The growth in health care expenses has fostered the development of many variations in methods of financing health services by payers seeking to limit their liability. The traditional fee-for-service approach, which utilizes a specific charge (set by the provider) for each service, is increasingly being replaced with other forms of reimbursement. The alternative methods used to compensate providers can be visualized as positioned along a continuum that reflects the relative magnitude of financial risk to the provider. At one extreme exists the fee-for-service option; at the other extreme is a capitation option whereby a flat fee is paid to providers to care for an individual irrespective of need. Under the traditional fee-for-service system, the only reimbursement-related risk for providers is that associated with setting charges at levels sufficient to cover service production costs. Conceptually, cost-based reimbursement systems carry the least amount of provider risk. In practice, however, reimbursement may be subject to cost caps and involve risk that is a function of the degree of consensus between provider and payer on what constitutes cost. Cost-containment efforts by payers have resulted in modifications to the fee-for-service system that increase financial risk to providers. Such modifications include negotiated fee discounts, establishment of reimbursement maximums for specific services, competitive bidding, limiting payment to some percentile of what other

area providers charge, and formal fixed-fee schedules that remu-
nerate participating providers at a rate that is usually the lower of
the provider's charge or the fee schedule amount.

At the opposite extreme of the risk continuum, payers seek to
bundle services and control volume with the objective of transferring all risk associated with volume and case-mix (distribution of
service types) increases to the provider, while controlling future
increases in payments. In this financing alternative the delivery
system, in essence, becomes the insurer. Capitation or premium is
the method of payment in this system. The payment rate is established for a specific time period during which the delivery system
is responsible for providing an agreed-upon package of medical
benefits to an individual or family based on their health care needs
and without regard to the volume or type of services needed.

Given the diverse nature of rural America, it is difficult to assess all
the implications of various payment systems for rural health care
providers. Nonetheless, it seems clear that incentives for the assumption of greater provider risk are frequently absent in rural systems. A
primary motivation in adopting payment systems with greater provider risk is a reduction in payer expense and/or risk. Incentives for
provider participation usually involve protection or enhancement of
the patient base and, in the case of capitation, a reasonable expectation that the participating provider's system can outperform the
pooled experience on which the payment rate was based, resulting in
a larger profit margin for those willing to accept the additional
volume risk. But providers in more sparsely populated areas have
less incentive than their urban counterparts to accept additional risks
to protect their patient base, which may be threatened more by a
decline in the local economy than by competing providers. In addition, if a provider's market share is already large, there is relatively
less to gain from an expanded share of patients. For example, organizations seeking discounts from hospitals have more success when
the discount can be justified by increased patient volume. Such justi-
fications are more difficult to achieve in areas where spatial monopo-
lies may already exist.

The Federal Government's Role

The federal government, as a major payer, has been very active
in introducing and facilitating the spread of alternative payment

systems. The impetus for these innovations has come from efforts to reduce the rate of growth in federally funded health care outlays. An example is the prospective payment system (PPS) for hospitals introduced into the Medicare system in 1983. Prior to 1983 cost-based reimbursement was the primary method of reimbursing hospitals under the Medicare program. However, by the early 1980s this payment system had became increasingly viewed as inherently inflationary. In 1983 a fundamental shift from cost-based reimbursement for hospital services to a per-case system was created as part of the Social Security legislation. The impact on the hospital industry was not uniform and the new system was thought by many to jeopardize the very survival of a significant segment of the rural hospital industry. Issues of inequitable treatment of rural hospitals were voiced by rural advocates, and the concern generated over the PPS legislation has been credited, along with a declining rural economy and concerns related to access to care, with heralding a new era of Congressional interest in rural health (Patton, 1989).

Increased sensitivity to rural health care systems has been instrumental in achieving rurally oriented modifications in PPS and in shaping the treatment of rural physicians under the currently evolving Medicare fee schedule. Ironically, many reforms propose a return to cost-based reimbursement for our most vulnerable rural health care institutions. Such reforms, however, continue to be tempered by concerns over the federal deficit. The current and future redistributional impacts on rural areas of these fundamental changes in the financing system should be documented, and the relationships among expenditure patterns, financing systems, delivery systems, utilization rates, and the health of local populations must be more fully understood in a rural context. Such information is essential to guide policy if rural health is to be maximized in an era in which interest is likely to remain focused on restraining health expenditures.

Issues in Geographic Variation in Medicare Expenditures

Prior to focusing on the geographic distribution of per capita Medicare expenditures, a number of specific observations relevant to Medicare expenditures in rural areas should be noted. Hospital reimbursement under PPS results in rural hospitals receiving less than their urban counterparts for the same service. The lower rural payments under PPS have been reported to be due to (1) a 40 percent difference in Medicare costs per case based on data from 1981 Medicare cost reports, and (2) Congressional concerns related to the rapid redistribution of funds that would occur under national rates (Special Committee on Aging, U.S. Senate, 1988). A report on the early experience under PPS notes that, during the early years, U.S. hospitals recorded profit levels above those of the 1970s, with a peak average total margin of 6.2 percent in 1984. However, even in the early years there were signs that smaller rural hospitals were in trouble. While 100 percent of the largest urban hospitals and 98.1 percent of major teaching hospitals had positive Medicare payment margins, only 67.8 percent of the smallest rural hospitals reported positive payment margins (Guterman et al., 1988). Falling operating margins and hospital closures, subsequent to the passage of PPS, increased pressure on Congress to reduce the rural/urban disparity and provide differential treatment for certain classes of rural hospitals. Legislative changes designed to strengthen the financial position of rural hospitals have been enacted since the third year of PPS; however, legislation throughout the latter half of the 1980s remained incremental in its approach to the rural/urban differential. The decade ended with advocates continuing to push for elimination of differential payments to rural hospitals while others raised concerns that rural hospital problems extended beyond PPS and Medicare (Prospective Payment Assessment Commission, 1989).

The traditional method of reimbursing physicians under Medicare has also led to geographic payment inequities. Researchers have noted large variations in prevailing and approved charges for physician services under the Medicare program (Office of Technology Assessment, U.S. Congress, 1986; Physician Payment Review Commission, 1988, 107). In their 1988 report to Congress, the Physician Payment Review Commission stated that charges are generally higher in urban areas but that the differences are often modest and primarily due to differences in practice expense. They concluded that "substantial geographic inequities do exist, but they lie more in the differences among specific urban or rural localities" (Physician Payment Review Commission, 1988, 108).

Medicare Financing

The Medicare program has two component parts. Part A (Hospital Insurance) covers short-term hospitalization, skilled nursing care, hospice care, and some home health services. Part B (Supplementary Medical Insurance) covers physician and ancillary services, hospital outpatient care, and some home health services. Revenues to support Part A are derived from Social Security payroll taxes assessed on covered employers, employees, and the self-employed. This tax is levied at the rate of 1.45 percent of wage and salary earnings up to a maximum of $125,000 in 1991. Part B is financed from direct premiums paid by program participants and from general tax revenues. In 1989, the taxpayer subsidy for Part B was an estimated $1,004 per beneficiary (U.S. General Accounting Office, 1989). The relationship between premium and general revenues has varied over time. Under the original law premiums paid for 50 percent of the cost; however, beginning in 1974 increases in premiums were tied to the percentage increase in Social Security payments, causing the proportion of costs paid by beneficiary premiums to fall over time. The Social Security Amendments of 1983 halted this decline and allowed premium increases in 1984 and 1985 at a rate sufficient to produce 25 percent of total program outlays from beneficiary premiums. In addition to tax and premium revenue, the Medicare program incorporates cost-sharing provisions under both Parts A and B. These provisions, in the form of deductibles and co-insurance, reduce the expense of the program through the direct addition of revenue and by reducing demand.

It is important to recognize from both a rural/urban and a local/regional policy perspective that the financing of private sector health care insurance differs markedly from that of Medicare. In traditional insurance models, insurers systematically modify their ratings and premiums to reflect differences in relative costs and utilization associated with providing services to identifiable groups. These groups are often defined on the basis of employer/industry affiliation or geographic criteria. Referred to as experience rating, this practice limits the interemployer and intergeographic effects of the insurance mechanism. Premium income reflects the utilization pattern of pool participants, the prevailing level of relevant health care costs, and the cost associated with administering the pool. It does not reflect the utilization of groups defined outside the pool or the cost of care in distant geographic areas.

In contrast, Medicare creates a single nationwide pool of beneficiaries whose care is financed with revenues primarily derived from the regressive Social Security tax and the moderately progressive income tax. These sources account for about 90 percent of total Medicare expenditures, with the remainder generated from Part B premiums. Neither tax revenues nor premium levels are adjusted for interregional differences in utilization patterns or health care costs. Instead, these rates are adjusted only for changes in total utilization and average costs across the nation as a whole. As a consequence the Medicare system redistributes resources intergenerationally from a working to a retired population, from higher to lower wage earners, and from the relatively healthy to the very sick.

Although this redistribution was necessary to achieve societal goals of improved access to health services for the elderly and disabled, the current financing methods may also have some less desirable characteristics, involving the redistribution of resources in a manner that may reduce access to health services for selected subpopulations. For example, although cost-sharing provisions introduce a "user" fee and are designed to reduce demand for service and encourage efficient use of the system, they may also disproportionately affect the health status of sick low-income populations (Brook et al., 1984).

The system Medicare employs to reimburse for physician and hospital services also provides the opportunity for the redistribution of financial resources in a way that is counterproductive to the achievement of societal goals of equitable access to medical services for all citizens. Prevailing and approved charges for physician services in the Medicare program exhibit tremendous variation (Physician Payment Review Commission, 1988, 108). These differentials, which are based on historical charging practices at the local level, cannot be adequately explained by differences in practice expense and/or differences in cost of living. A direct consequence is that local areas with historically high charges relative to cost are financed through the Medicare system in part by surcharges from areas with a historical record of charges that are low relative to costs. The effects of this redistribution are not limited to the Medicare population. Problems of resource reallocation under Medicare can be seen in the form of disproportionate expense to the non-Medicare population through cost shifting to other payers. Furthermore, the likelihood and/or magnitude of the cost shift increases with each reduction of federal payments under Medicare.

Documenting the current geographic distribution of Medicare expenditures is an important initial step in the process of assessing the implications of Medicare payment policies for rural health. A basic knowledge of the prevailing distribution of resources is useful in better understanding the potential for differential system impact. In addition, the actual distributional relationships themselves may be symptomatic of problems with the health care delivery system, including different levels of unmet need and/or demand, and differential payment levels and/or delivery system efficiencies. Finally, the absolute level of expenditures across different regions and other political subdivisions may itself have important ramifications for beneficiaries. This last point has particular relevance given research that indicates that higher per-beneficiary Medicare expenditures are associated with significantly lower mortality rates (Hadley, 1988).

Methodology

The distribution of Medicare resources in recent years was examined across different regions of the country and among different subdivisions of those regions. The county represented the basic unit of analysis but different definitions of rurality and urbanity were utilized to provide additional perspective on Medicare per capita expenditure variation. This additional insight is needed considering the diversity that exists among all counties, but particularly among nonmetropolitan counties. Adjusted average per capita costs (AAPCC) for aged Medicare beneficiaries were utilized to evaluate the prevailing distribution of Medicare resources under Part A and Part B.

The Office of the Actuary in the Health Care Financing Administration (HCFA) annually computes Part A and Part B AAPCCs for aged, disabled, and chronic renal beneficiaries. These rates, adjusted for age, sex, welfare, and institutional status, form the basis for monthly capitation payments to health maintenance organizations (HMOs) and competitive medical plans operating under risk contracts with HCFA. The rates are estimates of 95 percent of the federal government's per capita fee-for-service cost associated with provision of Medicare benefits to Medicare-eligible beneficiaries in a county (Palsbo, 1989). The 5-percent reduction reflects a mandatory "savings" to the federal government under the Medicare risk-contracting program. Since the AAPCC estimates only the government's expected per capita expenditures, it excludes beneficiary liabilities associated with deductibles, co-payments (currently 20 percent of approved Part B services), and balance-billed provider fees in excess of Medicare-approved levels.

AAPCCs are determined prospectively based on an estimate of the average federal monthly expenditures for Medicare-eligible beneficiaries in the United States, and a county-specific geographic adjustment. The annual national estimate is based on actual Medicare expenditures from the previous year and projections of changes in beneficiary eligibility, program scope, and payment amounts. For Part A, changes in the latter category are affected by factors such as increases in hospital labor and nonlabor prices, input intensity, and volume of service; for Part B, changes in the mix of services attributable to beneficiaries' aging, visits per enrollee, and the use of specialists and technologies influence payments. The county-specific geographic adjustment, which transforms the national estimate into its county-level equivalent, is based on historical differences between county and national per capita Medicare expenses. A five-year simple moving average of the ratio of county to national per capita expenditures is utilized in the geographic adjustment. This adjustment minimizes the effect annual variations in county per capita expense would otherwise have on HMO payment rates.

In addition to the geographic adjustment, counties with Medicare-eligible HMO enrollees require another adjustment that "nets out" the total federal cost of providing Medicare benefits to these enrollees. This adjustment reduces total estimated county Medicare expenditures by the amount paid to HMOs, leaving estimated fee-for-service expenditures as the residual. A similar adjustment to beneficiary numbers permits the estimation of per capita fee-for-service cost. This estimate reflects the government's expected average monthly fee-for-service expenditure associated with providing Medicare benefits to the *county's average beneficiary*. A final adjustment for demographic differences between the county's beneficiary population and the U.S. Medicare beneficiary population is made, and the resultant per capita expenditure is discounted 5 percent to yield the AAPCC.

The result of these adjustments is an estimate of 95 percent of the federal government's fee-for-service-equivalent, county per capita cost associated with providing Medicare benefits to the *average U.S. Medicare-eligible beneficiary* in a specific county. As an estimate of 95 percent of the monthly fee-for-service cost for Medicare beneficiaries for Part A and B, the AAPCC is an indicator of both the relative costs of services performed and the frequency and mix of those services at the county level for a standard demographic mix of beneficiaries.

Spatial Distributions

The geographic distribution of Medicare Part B AAPCCs (fig. 12.1) is strongly influenced by the physician component of Part B, which has comprised approximately 75 percent of all Part B expenditures in recent years. Counties ranking among the highest 20 percent of all counties are generally concentrated on the west coast, in Nevada and Arizona, along the upper east coast, and in Florida. Concentrated areas are also evident in the far western counties of Texas, the Gulf areas of Texas, and the industrial areas of eastern Michigan, northeastern Ohio, and Pennsylvania. Other county clusters with high rates include the Appalachian regions of West Virginia and eastern Kentucky, central and western Kansas, and areas in Arkansas, Colorado, and New Mexico. AAPCCs for these counties averaged $125.39 for 1989, about 19.5 percent more than the $104.91 average for all counties.

In contrast, the lowest 20 percent of the 1989 Part B AAPCCs are concentrated in the upper plains states, particularly Nebraska; large sections of Kentucky, South Carolina, Iowa, and Minnesota; eastern South Dakota; central Mississippi; northern Louisiana; western Virginia; and southern Missouri. AAPCCs in these counties averaged $59.98, or only 56 percent of the U.S. average.

The general pattern that emerges from an examination of fig. 12.1 is that the midwestern and southern regions of the country are overrepresented in the lower half of the AAPCC distribution and the west and northeast regions are overrepresented in the upper half. Average Part B rates are lower in the midwest ($91.83)

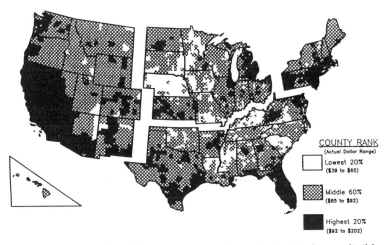

Fig. 12.1. Part B adjusted average per capita costs for Medicare-eligible aged beneficiaries (1989). Data were unavailable for Alaska.
Source: Office of the Actuary, U.S. Health Care Financing Administration.

and south ($95.97) than in the west ($129.10) and northeast ($113.69).

The higher rates in the west and northeast are reflected in higher AAPCCs for both metropolitan and nonmetropolitan counties in these regions. In the west, 76 percent of the counties ranked above the median U.S. rate, including all of the metropolitan counties and 70 percent of the nonmetropolitan counties. The situation was similar in the northeast, where 77 percent of the metropolitan counties and 63 percent of the nonmetropolitan counties were ranked in the upper half of the expenditure distribution.

A disproportionately large percentage of nonmetropolitan counties in the midwest and south were ranked below the U.S. median. Although 78 percent of the counties in the midwest and south are classified as nonmetropolitan, over 88 percent of the regions' counties below the U.S. median were nonmetropolitan.

Nationally, nonmetropolitan counties represented a disproportionately large share of the counties ranked below the U.S. median. Fifty-eight percent of all nonmetropolitan counties had Part B AAPCCs that fell under the U.S. median in 1989. This compares to only 24 percent of all metropolitan counties that were similarly positioned. Average rates were consistently

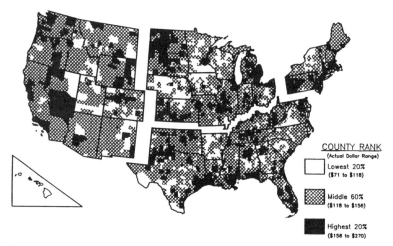

Fig. 12.2. Part A adjusted average per capita costs for Medicare-eligible
aged beneficiaries (1989). Data were unavailable for Alaska.
Source: Office of the Actuary, U.S. Health Care Financing Administration.

lower in nonmetropolitan counties as well. This basic relationship
was constant across regions and resulted in a nonmetropolitan
rate that averaged only 67.6 percent of the metropolitan rate across
the United States.

The distribution of 1989 Part A AAPCCs is depicted in fig. 12.2.
As was the case for Part B AAPCCs, the northeast coastal area; the
industrial areas of eastern Michigan, northern Ohio, and western
Pennsylvania; Florida; west Texas and the Texas Gulf coast area;
southwestern West Virginia and eastern Kentucky; and much of
Nevada appear among the highest expenditure areas. Clusters of
high-cost counties also are evident in the central and western
Dakotas, central Tennessee, southern and western Kansas, eastern
Wyoming, and parts of Oregon and Washington. AAPCCs averaged $185.76 in the counties in the highest 20 percent of the distri-
bution in 1989, about 17 percent more than the $158.81 average for
all counties.

Large portions of Nebraska, Iowa, Minnesota, Arkansas, Utah,
South Carolina, and New Mexico are included among the lowest
Part A reimbursed counties. In addition, significant sections in
upstate New York, western Virginia, Idaho, Montana, Wisconsin,
and Colorado are also in the lowest expenditure quintile. Counties

in the lowest 20 percent of the distribution averaged $109.23, or 69 percent of the U.S. average for Part A in 1989.

In general, there is a positive relationship between Part B and Part A AAPCCs. Thus, counties that have higher (lower) Part B expenditures also tend to have higher (lower) Part A expenditures per beneficiary. This basic relationship is reflected in the correlation coefficients between Part B and Part A expenditures, which ranged in value from .61 to .64 over the 1985–1989 period. Although these correlations are statistically significant, the size of the coefficients indicates that the relationship does not hold for many counties. Indeed, differences between Part A and Part B per capita expenditures are apparent in comparisons between figs. 12.1 and 12.2. In particular, it appears that Part A expenditures are relatively lower in large portions of California and Arizona compared to those under Part B. Conversely, generally higher Part A expenditures per beneficiary are evident in Missouri, Kentucky, Illinois, and areas in the southern region.

Average Part A expenditures were lowest in the south ($148.41), highest in the northeast ($173.12), and nearly equal in the midwest ($159.65) and west ($159.34). Metropolitan county averages were higher in all regions than corresponding nonmetropolitan average expenditures and resulted in a 28.8 percent difference in the average Part A expenditures for these counties. Metropolitan counties in the northeastern ($177.59) and midwestern ($176.47) regions had significantly higher Part A expenditures than in the south ($158.07) and west ($165.02).

In comparison, nonmetropolitan counties exhibited smaller regional variations in average Part A expenditures. Nonmetropolitan county rates were highest in the northeast ($136.37), followed by the west ($132.01), the south ($130.64), and finally the midwest ($129.96). Intraregional differences between metropolitan and nonmetropolitan areas were highest in the midwest, where average rates for metropolitan counties were 35.8 percent higher than nonmetropolitan averages.

Temporal Patterns

Changes in the distribution of Part A and Part B AAPCCs were reviewed from 1985 to 1989 to gain insights into the temporal effects of policy initiatives, such as the institution of the PPS for hospitals. Whereas only modest changes were observed in the Part B distributions, changes in the distribution of Part A AAPCCs from 1985 to 1989 were clearly evident. In particular, the northeast, west, and midwest experienced general downward shifts in their Part A distributions while the south experienced an upward shift during this period. As a result of these changes, the south experienced a net increase of 185 counties in the upper half of the distribution in 1989 compared to 1985 levels. Approximately two-thirds of these were nonmetropolitan counties. This shift of government resources to the south was anticipated and resulted largely from the methodology used to estimate standardized payments in the hospital payment algorithm.

The mix between metropolitan and nonmetropolitan counties in the top half of the distribution also changed significantly in this period. The proportion of metropolitan counties increased from 32.7 percent to 37.1 percent, primarily as a result of more south region metropolitan counties ranking above the median in 1989. The number of metropolitan counties in the west and northeast ranked above the median also increased over the period. Nonmetropolitan counties in the midwest region were most affected by this shift. Of the total of 166 midwest counties that shifted from above-median Part A expenditures in 1985 to below-median expenditures in 1989, 163 were nonmetropolitan counties.

Nonmetropolitan County Type Differences

An analysis of the prevailing distribution of Medicare resources among different types of nonmetropolitan counties can provide additional insights into the differences that exist among these counties. This is an important activity particularly since most analyses of Medicare expenditures that focus on rural/urban differences treat nonmetropolitan counties (and metropolitan for that matter) as homogeneous elements for analysis. The heterogeneous nature of nonmetropolitan counties requires analyses that extend beyond a dichotomous rural/urban framework.

A number of nonmetropolitan county classification formats have been developed by both governmental agencies and other interests over the past twenty years in attempts to describe the underlying nature of nonmetropolitan county-level geopolitical

units (see chapter 2 and Hewitt, 1989). These efforts have generally utilized one of two basic approaches in developing their
classification scheme. They have either classified counties
based on their dominant aggregate economic activity or developed a classification format that utilizes a combination of geographic proximity to metropolitan areas, population size
and/or density, and/or intercounty worker commuting patterns. Although their conceptual frameworks are different, they
all seek a common goal: an improved understanding of the
impacts of policy initiatives on rural America. In the present
context, classification formats will be utilized for decomposing
nonmetropolitan counties into more meaningful mutually exclusive subgroups for analyzing the current distribution of
Medicare expenditures. The objective is a more complete understanding of the potential distributional impacts of Medicare
expenditures on rural beneficiaries and rural health care delivery systems. An implicit assumption in this analysis is that the
classification subgroups each represent a more homogeneous
collection of counties than the next higher level of classification,
which is metropolitan/nonmetropolitan.

Economic Classification Criteria

The economic classification system developed for the U.S.
Department of Agriculture (USDA) by Bender et al. provides
insight into the intrarural variations that currently exist in
Medicare expenditures per beneficiary. In terms of total Medicare expenditures (Part A and Part B), counties designated as
persistent poverty areas and counties highly dependent on
farming and related agricultural activities had much lower average per-beneficiary Medicare expenditures than other nonmetropolitan counties (Bender et al., 1985). Poverty counties'
expenditures averaged only 90.5 percent of the nonmetropolitan average expenditure per beneficiary in 1989 and farming
counties averaged 95.5 percent of the nonmetropolitan average
expenditure of $212.20 (table 12.1).

Conversely, counties dependent on mining activities and those
designated as retirement counties had significantly higher average per-beneficiary expenditure rates. These two county types had
average expenditures that were 9.8 percent and 5 percent above

Table 12.1. Distribution of Total AAPCCs by USDA County Economic Type (National Quartiles, 1989)

| County type[a] | Total | | Quartile | | | | | | | |
| | | | First (lowest) | | Second | | Third | | Fourth (highest) | |
	No. of counties	Mean[b] ($)	No. of counties	Mean ($)	No. of counties	Mean ($)	No. of counties	Mean ($)	No. of counties	Mean ($)
Metropolitan	626	287.57	36	181.40	86	201.01	159	224.19	345	304.28
Nonmetropolitan										
Farming	477	202.83	183	172.80	115	200.84	103	222.84	76	262.95
Federal lands	42	215.16	5	178.42	10	201.71	20	222.63	7	267.16
Manufacturing	437	208.64	137	176.35	131	200.19	111	223.92	58	258.16
Mining	110	233.04	10	182.53	24	199.66	30	223.99	46	265.66
Poverty	43	192.11	20	170.46	12	201.47	9	224.85	2	244.19
Retirement	178	222.78	34	179.19	57	199.78	57	224.42	30	258.49
Special government	112	213.58	25	173.42	35	200.72	34	224.46	18	252.92
Multiclass[c]	674	214.87	194	177.11	199	200.40	155	225.57	126	262.02
Unclassified[d]	370	208.47	118	178.41	107	199.45	88	221.64	57	262.99
Nonmetropolitan total	2,443	212.20	726	176.37	690	200.17	607	223.99	420	260.48

[a]Classification is based on criteria developed by Bender et al. for the Agriculture and Rural Development Division, Economic Research Service, USDA.
[b]Weighted by estimated aged beneficiary population.
[c]Counties that met more than one subgroup classification criterion.
[d]Counties that did not meet minimum subgroup classification standards.

the nonmetropolitan average, respectively. However, although these counties had high expenditures relative to all nonmetropolitan counties, each was more than 10 percent below the U.S. average of $264.06 in 1989.

There is a relatively consistent pattern in the expenditure rankings of different types of nonmetropolitan counties over the 1985–1989 period. Poverty and farming counties have been consistently ranked as the two lowest nonmetropolitan county types on this basis, whereas retirement and mining counties consistently have been ranked as the highest nonmetropolitan expenditure counties. Farming counties' relative expenditure rate remained nearly constant at about 77 percent of the U.S. average over the 1985–1989 period. Poverty counties increased their relative expenditure rate from 63.5 percent of the U.S. average in 1985 to 72.8 percent in 1989. Similarly, mining counties increased from 81.9 to 88.3 percent of the countrywide average.

Poverty and farming-dependent counties had the two lowest average Medicare expenditure rates for both Part A and Part B coverage. Poverty county Medicare beneficiaries' average Part A expenditures were about 96 percent of the nonmetropolitan average and 79.8 percent of the U.S. average in 1989. For Part B services, poverty county Medicare beneficiaries had an average per capita expenditure rate of $65.19, only 82 percent of the nonmetropolitan average and 62 percent of the U.S. average. Farming-dependent counties' Part A expenditures were only 88 percent of the U.S. average and their Part B expenditures were 69 percent of the U.S. average.

Mining-dependent counties ranked highest among nonmetropolitan counties in Part A and second highest in Part B average expenditures in 1989. Although these counties' Part A average was 11 percent greater than the nonmetropolitan average of $132.72, it was 7 percent less than the U.S. average.

Both regional and county type effects are apparent in the distribution of Medicare expenditures in 1989. The low ranking of poverty counties in terms of average total Medicare expenditures per beneficiary is almost exclusively a southern region phenomenon. A similar, although less extreme, effect is evident among farming counties: midwestern counties with low average expenditures have a significant downward effect on the total for all farming counties.

Metropolitan Proximity Criteria

An alternative to the economically based county classification is one based on urbanization and metropolitan proximity. Data displayed in table 12.2 are categorized on the basis of just such a system (McGranahan et al., 1986). The classification subgroups are defined to differentiate between the potential effects of direct (reflected in urban population) and indirect (reflected in metropolitan proximity) urbanization effects. Different population size groups are established to differentiate counties further on the basis of their urban populations and serve as proxies for unmeasured socioeconomic and demographic characteristics that are presumably highly correlated with urban population within these size groups.

The data in table 12.2 suggest a relatively consistent pattern of average total Medicare expenditures per beneficiary across metropolitan adjacent and nonadjacent counties and among counties with different urban population bases. Counties in the most populous metropolitan areas consistently have significantly higher per-beneficiary expenditures than either their smaller metropolitan counterparts or nonmetropolitan counties. These counties had average expenditures in 1989 that were 18.7 percent higher than the U.S. average, 28.8 percent higher than those for metropolitan counties with fewer than one million persons, and 49.7 percent higher than the nonmetropolitan county average. Data from 1985 and 1987 yield similar results, although the differences between the largest metropolitan counties and other counties have narrowed slightly.

Nonmetropolitan counties adjacent to metropolitan areas have consistently higher average expenditures per Medicare beneficiary than the corresponding nonadjacent counties in all years (table 12.2). In addition, nonmetropolitan counties with urban populations in excess of 20,000 persons have consistently higher adjacent-county and nonadjacent-county average expenditures than smaller nonmetropolitan counties. Clearly, proximity to a metropolitan county and urban population base affect the distribution of total Medicare expenditures.

Differences between the relative distributions of Part A and Part B Medicare expenditures were evident across the urban population/ metropolitan proximity continuum. In general, the percentage differences in average expenditures between county classification sub-

Table 12.2. Weighted[a] Average Total AAPCCs by Metropolitan/
Nonmetropolitan Designation, Metropolitan/Urban Population, and
Geographic Location (Selected Years)

Classification	No. of counties	Mean ($) 1985	Mean ($) 1987	Mean ($) 1989
Metropolitan[b]	713	210.78	228.28	284.48
Population over one million	227	235.10	252.34	313.29
Population under one million	486	175.93	193.79	243.18
Nonmetropolitan	2,361	151.09	163.73	209.30
Urban population over 20,000	287	157.44	169.51	216.26
Adjacent to metropolitan county	137	159.95	171.19	218.70
Not adjacent to metropolitan county	150	154.13	167.28	213.05
Urban population of 2,500–20,000	1,300	148.03	160.88	206.28
Adjacent to metropolitan county	551	150.28	163.51	209.53
Not adjacent to metropolitan county	749	145.87	158.35	203.15
Rural[c]	774	149.02	162.12	205.61
Adjacent to metropolitan county	228	149.32	165.70	210.65
Not adjacent to metropolitan county	546	148.85	160.04	202.68
Total	3,074[d]	194.51	210.68	263.99

[a]AAPCCs weighted by estimated aged beneficiary population.

[b]This classification is based on total metropolitan statistical area (MSA) population rather than county population. County totals represent the number of counties defined within MSAs whose total population exceeds (or is less than) one million persons.

[c]Includes both completely rural counties (i.e., counties with no urban population) and counties that are primarily rural but share an urban population with an adjacent county. In the latter, the urban population is less than 2,500 persons in the rural-designated county.

[d]Of the thirty-nine counties missing, one is in Hawaii and the other thirty-eight are independent cities in Virginia.

groups were smaller for Part A than for Part B. For example, the difference between large metropolitan counties' average Part A expenditures and the U.S. average Part A expenditures was 15 percent, compared to 23.4 percent for Part B, in 1989. The difference in average 1989 Part A expenditures between large metropolitan counties and nonmetropolitan counties was 39.8 percent, compared to a 66.3-percent difference between Part B expenditures.

Differences also are apparent among nonmetropolitan counties with respect to Part A and Part B average expenditures. There appears to be less interclassification group variation in average expenditures for Part A than for Part B. The difference between the nonmetropolitan Part A average expenditure in 1989 ($131.33) and the highest nonmetropolitan subgroup average of $134.41 is only 2.3 percent and the difference between the highest and lowest average expenditures is only 4.3 percent. These differences are substantially less than the corresponding 11.6-percent and 21.4-percent differences for nonmetropolitan Part B expenditures.

A regional disaggregation of the data for 1989 reveals patterns very similar to those found in the economic classification format and in the simple metropolitan/nonmetropolitan classification. Nonmetropolitan midwestern counties are consistently either the lowest-average-expenditure counties or the second lowest in total expenditures and Part B expenditures across all regions and county classifications. Conversely, the western region consistently has the highest or the second highest average expenditure for total and Part B. The northeast is consistently high across county types for Part A.

Summary of Results

Medicare expenditures per beneficiary vary widely among different regions of the country, between metropolitan and nonmetropolitan counties, and even within the class of counties commonly referred to as "rural." It is important to recognize that some variation in expenditures per beneficiary is to be expected. Observed variation may reflect differences in the underlying need/demand for health care services by the elderly, differential reimbursements for services, and differences in the availability and accessibility of medical services in local areas. However, it is also important to recognize that large, consistent differences in the level of expenditures per beneficiary may be indicative of a system that performs poorly with respect to providing all beneficiaries equitable levels of service and may not be reimbursing all medical care providers on an equitable basis.

The general patterns observed in Medicare expenditures can be summarized as follows:

- Metropolitan counties have higher average expenditures per beneficiary than nonmetropolitan counties for services provided under Part A, under Part B, and in total. In percentage terms, the differences are smaller for Part A than Part B, but still amount to an average expenditure difference per beneficiary of about 29 percent for Part A. Average Part B expenditure differences were nearly 48 percent in 1989.
- Regional differences are apparent in the distribution of Medicare expenditures. The northeastern and western regions have higher average Part B expenditures than the midwest and south. This relationship is relatively consistent across both metropolitan and nonmetropolitan counties within the respective regions. Average expenditures for Part B services are much lower in the nonmetropolitan counties in the midwest and south than elsewhere.
- Part A regional differences also exist but are different from those observed for Part B. In particular, the midwest's Part A average is much higher relative to the U.S. average than that for Part B. Conversely, the west's average is much lower relative to the U.S. average for Part A than for Part B.
- Among nonmetropolitan counties there is a relatively stable pattern of expenditures across different county classes. Poverty and farming-dependent counties have consistently the two lowest average expenditures among nonmetropolitan counties across all three expenditure measures for the time periods analyzed. Mining-dependent counties and those designated as retirement counties were consistently ranked as the highest-average-expenditure counties.
- Among nonmetropolitan counties, average Part B and total expenditures were higher in metropolitan adjacent counties than in nonadjacent counties in all years examined. Average Part A expenditures demonstrated a similar but less consistent pattern. Significantly higher average expenditures were noted in nonmetropolitan counties with larger urban population bases.

Discussion

There are many potential reasons for the observed spatial variation in Medicare per capita expenditures. These include geographic variation in physician and hospital payment rates,
geographic differences in the need and demand for medical care,
regional differences in the supply of health care providers and
institutions, and differences in the practice style of local medical
communities. A significant part of the variation in per capita
Medicare expenditures for Part B services has been shown to be
due to geographic variation in Medicare payments to physicians
(Schmelzer, 1990), and it is likely that the differences in hospital
reimbursement, embodied in PPS, also contribute to regional variation in Medicare per capita expenditures under Part A. A key
issue being considered by the Prospective Payment Assessment
Commission and the Physician Payment Review Commission
(groups that advise Congress on issues related to Part A and Part
B of Medicare) is the extent to which geographic variation in
Medicare reimbursement is justified on the basis of differences in
input costs beyond the control of local hospitals and physicians
providing the service. To the extent that variation in payment is
not explained by such input cost differences, justification of residual differentials is difficult.

The impact of need and demand factors on the variation in
Medicare per capita expenditures is difficult to isolate. Some of
these effects are controlled for by standardizing per capita rates by
the age, sex, welfare, and institutional status of the Medicare beneficiary. However, there is also evidence of geographic variation in
injury and illness rates within specific age and sex cohorts that
would not be accounted for in this standardization. Hence such
variation almost certainly contributes to the observed differences
in Medicare per capita expenditures. Other influences may stem
from geographic variation in factors that influence demand. Evidence from the literature points to reduced demand for medical
care with increased cost sharing (Manning et al., 1988). Although
the quantitative implications of this finding for differences in
Medicare per capita costs are unclear, a number of authors have
commented on the depressive effect of cost sharing on access to or
utilization of services in elderly populations (Nelson et al., 1989;
Sorkin, 1986; Yett et al., 1983). The Medicare benefit package itself
was designed to incorporate cost sharing provisions in an effort to

limit demand for services. Given these relationships, geographic variation in access to physicians who accept assignment and/or regional variation in the purchase of medigap insurance by beneficiaries may influence the observed findings.

The availability and accessibility of services also has a direct impact on utilization and expenditures. These relationships have been explored by researchers studying the distance decay effects in medical care (McGuirk and Porrell, 1984; Mayer, 1983). Such work has particular relevance to rural areas and to health policymakers interested in insuring equitable access to basic health services for all Medicare beneficiaries. Although the role of Medicare financing policies in the distribution of physicians and hospitals is not fully understood, Congress is already struggling with reforms to insure the survival of vulnerable rural hospitals by experimenting with concepts such as essential access facilities. While new technologies continue to bring more sophisticated services to rural populations, studies are progressing on the relationship of patient outcomes and volume of service. Results from these studies will help to determine the future scope of services delivered on site in rural areas versus those that many rural residents will have to travel to obtain.

Finally, there is a renewed interest in small-area-variation studies and studies of the effect that physician practice style has on expenditure patterns and health outcomes. Techniques and methodologies developed in such studies may ultimately be helpful in better defining the scope and geographic distribution of services needed to maximize the health of rural populations.

References

Abler, R., Adams, J. S., and Gould, P. 1971. *Spatial organization: The geographer's view of the world*. Englewood Cliffs, New Jersey: Prentice-Hall.

Abrahamson, J. 1980. Types of rural communities. In *Rural social work forum conference proceedings*, ed. W. Shera. Victoria, British Columbia, Canada: University of Victoria.

Adams, O. 1989. Canada's doctors—Who they are and what they do: Lessons from the CMA's 1986 manpower survey. *Canadian Medical Association Journal* 140:212–221.

Aiken, L. H., Lewis, C. E., Craig, J., Mendenhall, R. C., Blendon, R. J., and Rogers, D. E. 1979. The contribution of specialists to the delivery of primary care. *New England Journal of Medicine* 300:1363–1370.

Airola, T. M., and Parker, R. A. 1983. Population redistribution within the rural-urban fringe: A typology of small town and rural municipalities in the state of New Jersey. *Environment and Planning A* 15:1457–1474.

American College of Emergency Physicians. 1987. Guidelines for trauma care systems. *Annals of Emergency Medicine* 16(4):459–463.

———. 1988a. Prehospital advanced life support skills, medications and equipment. *Annals of Emergency Medicine* 17(10):1109–1111.

———. 1988b. Guidelines for emergency medical services systems. *Annals of Emergency Medicine* 17(7):742–745.

American College of Surgeons. Committee on Trauma. 1986. Hospital resources documents: Field categorization of trauma patients (field triage). *Bulletin of the American College of Surgeons* 71(10):17–21.

———. Committee on Trauma. 1987. *Hospital and prehospital resources for optimal care of the injured patient*. Chicago: American College of Surgeons.

American Hospital Association. 1987. *Environmental assessment for rural hospitals 1988*. Chicago: American Medical Association.

———. 1989. *Rural hospital closure: Management and community implications*. Chicago: Hospital Research and Educational Trust.

American Institutes for Research. 1990. *Evaluation of the impact of the National Area Health Education Center Program*. Final report, Contract No. 240-88-0031. Rockville, Maryland: Division of Medicine, Bureau of Health Professions.

American Medical Association. 1971. *Directory of approved internships and residencies 1971–1972*. Chicago: American Medical Association.

———. 1975. *Physician distribution and medical licensure in the U.S., 1974*, and *Special tabulations*. Chicago: American Medical Association, Center for Health Services Research and Development.

American Public Health Association. 1989. The nation's health. *State health notes* 19(11):24.

Amundson, B. A., and Rosenblatt, R. A. 1988. The rural hospital project: Conceptual background and current status. *Journal of Rural Health* 4:119–138.

Anderson, M., and Rosenberg, M. 1990. Ontario's Underserviced Area Program revisited: An indirect analysis. *Social Science and Medicine* 30: 35–44.

Anderson, P. B., Neuman, K. J., and Trimble, G. R. 1986. Trauma in the country: A statewide approach to trauma skills training for rural EMTs. *Journal of Emergency Medical Services* 11(3):61–62, 64.

Arizona Statewide Health Coordinating Council. 1985. *Primary care services in underserved areas.* In *Arizona state health plan 1985–1990*, pp. 8.1–8.46. Phoenix: Arizona Department of Health Services.

Arriaga, E. E. 1984. Measuring and explaining the change in life expectancies. *Demography* 21(1):83–92.

Babbott, D., Baldwin, D. C., Jolly, P., and Williams, D. J. 1988. The stability of early specialty preferences among U.S. medical school graduates in 1983. *Journal of the American Medical Association* 259:1970–1975.

Bagley, C., and MacDonald, M. 1984. Adult mental health sequels of child sexual abuse, physical abuse and neglect in maternally separated children. *Canadian Journal of Community Mental Health* 3:15–26.

Baker, S. P., Whitfield, M. S., and O'Neill, B. 1987. Geographic variations in mortality from motor vehicle crashes. *New England Journal of Medicine* 316:1384–1387.

―――. 1988. County mapping of injury mortality. *Journal of Trauma* 28(6): 741–745.

Baker, T. 1988. *Health personnel planning.* In *Health planning for effective management*, ed. W.A. Reinke, pp. 147–155. New York: Oxford University Press.

Bashshur, R. L., Shannon, G. W., and Metzner, C. A. 1971. Some ecological differentials in the use of medical services. *Health Services Research* 6:61–75.

Bass, R. L., and Paulman, P. M. 1983. The rural preceptorship as a factor in the residency selection: The Nebraska experience. *Journal of Family Practice* 17(4):716–719.

Beale, C. L. 1984. Poughkeepsie's complaint or defining metropolitan areas. *American Demographics* 6:29–48.

Beale, C. L., and Fuguitt, G. V. 1985. *Metropolitan and nonmetropolitan population growth in the United States since 1980.* CDE Working Paper 85-6. Madison, Wisconsin: Center for Demography and Ecology, University of Wisconsin-Madison.

Bean, E. 1988. Small rural hospitals struggle for survival under Medicare setup; Payment system exacerbates their passel of problems. *Wall Street Journal* January 4:1, 8.

Bell, M. 1980. Preparing social students for work in resource regions: The role of the urban university in teaching the study of human environments. In *Rural social work forum conference proceedings*, ed. W. Shera, pp. 41–65. Victoria, British Columbia, Canada: University of Victoria.

Belsky, J. 1980. Child maltreatment: An ecological integration. *American Psychologist* 35:320–325.

Bender, L. D., Green, B. L., Hady, T. F., Kuehn, J. A., Nelson, M. K., Parkinson, L. B., and Ross, P. J. 1985. *The diverse social and economic structure of nonmetropolitan America.* Economic Research Service, U.S. Department of Agriculture. Rural Development Research Report No. 49. Washington, D.C.: U.S. Government Printing Office.

Bennett, E. M. 1985. Native persons: An assessment of their relationship to the dominant culture and challanges for change. In *Theoretical and empirical advances in community mental health,* ed. E. M. Bennett and B. Tefft, pp. 53–63. Queenston, New York: Edwin Mellen.

Bennett, R. J. 1980. *The geography of public finance. Welfare under fiscal federalism and local government finance.* London: Methuen.

Ben-Sira, Z. 1983. The structure of a hospital's image. *Medical Care* 21:943–954.

Berk, M., Cafferata, G., and Hagan, M. 1984. Persons with limitations of activity: Health insurance, expenditures and use of services. In *NCHES Data Preview 19.* Washington, D.C.: National Center for Health Services Research.

Berk, M., Bernstein, A., and Taylor, A. 1983. The use and availability of medical care in health shortage areas. *Inquiry* 20:369–380.

Berry, B. J., and Garrison, W. L. 1958. A note on central place theory and the range of a good. *Economic Geography* 34:304–311.

Beyrouti, M., and Dion, M. 1990. *Focus on Canada: Canada's farm population.* Ottawa: Supply and Services Canada.

Bible, B. L. 1970. Physicians' views on medical practice in non-metropolitan areas. *Public Health Reports* 85:11–17.

Biklen, D. 1988. The myth of clinical judgement. *Journal of Social Issues* 44:127–140.

Bindman, A. B. 1989. *A public hospital closes: Impact on patients' access to care and health status.* Paper presented to the national meeting of the Robert Wood Johnson Clinical Scholars Program, November 6.

Bisbee, G. E., Jr., ed. 1982. *Management of rural primary care, concepts and cases.* Chicago: Hospital Research and Educational Trust, American Hospital Association.

Blondell, R., Smith, I., Byrne, M., and Higgins, C. W. 1989. Rural health, family practice, and Area Health Education Centers: A national study. *Family Medicine* 21(3):183–186.

Bohland, J. R., and Rowles, G. D. 1988. The significance of elderly migration to changes in elderly population concentration in the United States: 1960–1980. *Journal of Gerontology* 43:145–152.

Bonnen, J. T. 1988. *The statistical data base for rural America,* No. 88-80. East Lansing, Michigan: Department of Agricultural Economics, Michigan State University.

Bowe, F. 1980. *Rehabilitating America.* New York: Harper & Row.

Boyd, D. D., Edlich, R. F., and Micik, S. 1983. *Systems approach to emergency medical care.* Norwalk, Connecticut: Appleton-Century-Crofts.

Boyd, E. W., Konrad, T. R., and Seipp, C. 1982. In and out of the mainstream: The miner's medical program, 1946–78. *Journal of Public Health Policy* 3(4):432–444.

Boyle, M. H., Offord, D. R., Hoffman, H. G., Catlin, G. P., Byles, J. A., Cadman, D. T., Crawford, J. W., Links, P. S., Rae-Grant, N., and Szatmari, P. 1987. Ontario child health study: I. Methodology. *Archives of General Psychiatry* 44:826–831.

Bradham, D. D., McLaughlin, C. P., and Ricketts, T. C. 1985. The ability of aggregate data to predict self-sufficiency levels in subsidized rural primary care practices. *Journal of Rural Health* 1(2):56–68.

Brearley, W. D., Simpson, W., and Baker, R. M. 1982. Family practice as a specialty choice: Effect of pre-medical and medical education. *Journal of Medical Education* 57:449–454.

Brink, S. 1984. *Inventory of programs in Canada for housing the elderly living independently.* Ottawa: Canada Mortgage and Housing Corporation.

Bronfenbrenner, U. 1977. Toward an experimental ecology of human development. *American Psychologist* 32:513–531.

———. 1986. Ecology of the family as a context for human development: Research perspectives. *Developmental Psychology* 22:723–742.

Brook, R., Ware, J., Rogers, W., Keeler, E., Daves, A., Sherbourne, C., Goldberg, G., Lohr, K., Camp, P., and Newhouse, J. 1984. The effect of coinsurance on the health of adults. Results from the Rand Health Insurance Experiment. Rand Health Insurance Experiment Series. Santa Monica, California: Rand Corporation.

Brown, D. L., and Beale, C. L. 1981. Diversity in post-1970 population trends. In *Nonmetropolitan America in transition*, ed. A. H. Hawley and S. M. Mazie, pp. 27–71. Chapel Hill, North Carolina: University of North Carolina Press.

Bryant, E. S., and El-Attar, M. 1984. Migration and redistribution of the elderly: A challenge to community services. *Gerontologist* 24:634–640.

Burfield, W. B., Hough, D. E., and Marder, W. D. 1986. Location of medical education and choice of location of practice. *Journal of Medical Education* 61(7):545–554.

Burkhauser, R. V., and Havemen, R. H. 1982. *Disability and work. The economics of American policy.* Baltimore: Johns Hopkins University Press.

Butler, M. 1991. Population Section, Economic Research Service, U.S. Department of Agriculture, Washington, D.C. Personal communication, August 5.

Butler, P. A. 1988. *Too poor to be sick.* APHA Public Policy Series. Washington, D.C.: American Public Health Association.

Butter, I., Wright, G., and Tasca, D. 1978. FMGs in Michigan: A case of dependence. *Inquiry* 15:45–57.

Cales, R. H. 1984. Trauma mortality in Orange County: The effect of implementation of a regional trauma system. *Annals of Emergency Medicine* 13(1):15–24.

Cales, R. H., and Trunkey, D. D. 1985. Preventable trauma deaths. *Journal of the American Medical Association* 254(8):1059–1063.

Calkins, B. M. 1987. Life-style and chronic disease in western society. In *Public health and the environment: The United States experience*, ed. M. R. Greenberg, pp. 25–75. New York: Guilford Press.

Canadian Association of Schools of Social Work. 1976. *Social work education for practice in rural and northern regions.* Winnipeg, Manitoba, Canada: Canadian Association of Schools of Social Work.

Carlson, E. D. 1984. Social determinants of low birth weight in a high-risk population. *Demography* 21(2):207–215.

Carnegie Council on Policy Studies in Higher Education. 1976. *Progress and problems in medical and dental education: Federal support versus federal control.* San Francisco: Jossey-Bass.

Carter, G. M., Chu, D. S., Koehler, J. E., Slighton, R. L., and Williams, A. P., Jr. 1974. *Federal manpower legislation and the academic health centers: An interim report*. Report No. R1464-HEW. Santa Monica, California: Rand Corporation.

Castellani, P. J. 1987. *The political economy of developmental disabilities*. Baltimore: Paul H. Brookes.

Catalano, R. 1979. *Health, behaviour and the community*. New York: Pergamon.

Catalano, R., and Dooley, D. 1977. Economic predictors of depressed mood and stressful life events in a metropolitan community. *Journal of Health and Social Behavior* 18:292–307.

———. 1979. The economy as stressor: A sectoral analysis. *Review of Social Economy* 37:175–187.

Certo, T. F., Rogers, F. B., and Pilcher, D. B. 1983. Review of care of fatally injured patients in a rural state: 5-year follow-up. *Journal of Trauma* 23(7):559–565.

Champion, D. J., and Olsen, D. 1971. Physician behavior in southern Appalachia: Some recruitment factors. *Journal of Health and Social Behavior* 12:245–252.

Champion, H. R., and Mabee, M. S. 1990. An American crisis in trauma care reimbursement. *Emergency Care Quarterly* July:65–87.

Champion, H. R., Sacco, W. J., Hannan, D. S., Lepper, R. L., Atzinger, E. S., Copes, W. S., and Prall, R. S. 1980. Assessment of injury severity: The triage index. *Critical Care Medicine* 8(4):201–208.

Champion, H. R., Sacco, W. J., Carnazzo, A. J., Copes, W., and Fouty, W. J. 1981. Trauma score. *Critical Care Medicine* 9(9):672–676.

Champion, H. R., Sacco, W. J., and Copes, W. S. 1991. Trauma scoring. In *Trauma*, Second Edition, ed. E. E. Moore, K. L. Mattox, and D. V. Feliciano, pp. 23–33. East Norwalk, Connecticut: Appleton & Lange.

Chappell, N. L. 1987. Canadian income and health care policy: Implications for the elderly. In *Aging in Canada: Social perspectives*, Second Edition, ed. V. Marshall, pp. 489–504. Toronto: Fitzhenry and Whiteside.

Chappell, N. L., and Penning, M. 1979. The trend away from institutionalization: Humanism or economic efficiency? *Research on Aging* 1:361–387.

Chappell, N. L., Strain, L. A., and Blandford, A. A. 1986. *Aging and health care: A social perspective*. Toronto: Holt, Rinehart & Winston.

Christaller, W. 1933. Die zentralen Orte in Süddeutschland. Jena, Germany: Gustav Fischer Verlag.

Christianson, J. B., and Faulkner, L. 1981. The contribution of rural hospitals to local economies. *Inquiry* 18:46–60.

Ciriacy, E. W., Bland, C. J., Stoller, J. E., and Prestwood, J. S. 1980. Graduate follow-up in the University of Minnesota affiliated hospitals residency training program in family practice and community health. *Journal of Family Practice* 11(5):719–730.

Clifford, W. B., Heaton, T. B., Lichter, D. T., and Fuguitt, G. V. 1983. Components of change in the age composition of nonmetropolitan America. *Rural Sociology* 48(3):458–470.

Coleman, S. 1976. *Physician distribution and rural access to medical services: Executive summary*. Report prepared for DHEW, HRA, Division of Medicine, Contract No. 231-750-0613, Report No. R-1887/1. Santa Monica, California: Rand Corporation.

Collier, K. 1984. *Social work with rural peoples: Theory and practice*. Vancouver, British Columbia, Canada: New Star Books.

Conger, R. D., McCarty, J. A., Yang, R. K., Lahey, B. B., and Kropp, J. P. 1984. Perception of child, child-rearing values, and emotional distress as mediating links between environmental stressors and observed maternal behaviour. *Child Development* 55:2234–2247.

Connidis, I. 1985. The service needs of older people: Implications for public policy. *Canadian Journal on Aging* 1:3–10.

Cooper, J. K., Heald, K. A., and Samuels, M. 1972. The decision for rural practice. *Journal of Medical Education* 47:939–944.

Cooper, J. K., Heald, K. A., Samuels, M., and Coleman, S. 1975. Rural or urban practice: Factors influencing the location decision of primary care physicians. *Inquiry* 12:18–25.

Cordes, S. M. 1987. *The changing rural environment and the relationship between health services and rural development.* Commissioned paper prepared for the Rural Health Services Agenda Conference, San Diego, California, December 13–15.

———. 1989. The changing rural environment and the relationship between health services and rural development. *Health Services Research* 23(6):757–784.

Cosgrove, D. 1987. New directions in cultural geography. *Area* 19:95–101.

Cottington, E. M., Young, J. C., Shufflebarger, C. M., Kyes, F., Peterson, F. V., Jr., and Diamons, D. L. 1988. The utility of physiological status, injury site, and injury mechanism in identifying patients with major trauma. *Journal of Trauma* 28(3):305–311.

Coudroglou, A., and Poole, D. L. 1984. *Disability, work and social policy. Models for social welfare.* New York: Springer-Verlag.

Coward, R. T. 1979. Planning community services for the rural elderly: Implications for research. *Gerontologist* 19:275–282.

Cromartie, J. 1990. *Black long distance migration to the United States South, 1975–80: A comparison of metropolitan and non-metropolitan destinations.* Unpublished Ph.D. dissertation, Department of Geography, University of North Carolina at Chapel Hill.

Cromley, E. K. 1989. *The impact of the National Health Service Corps program on physician availability in urban and rural areas.* Paper presented to the 12th Annual Applied Geography Conference, Binghamton, New York, October 19.

Crowley, A. E., Etzel, S. I., and Shaw, H. A. 1987. Graduate medical education in the United States. *Journal of the American Medical Association* 258(8):1031–1040.

Crown, W. H. 1988. State economic implications of elderly interstate migration. *Gerontologist* 28:533–539.

Dahmann, D. 1989. Population Division, Bureau of the Census, U.S. Department of Commerce, Washington, D.C. Personal communication, May.

Dahms, F. A. 1987. *Population migration and the elderly: Ontario 1971–1981.* Occasional Paper No. 9. Guelph, Ontario, Canada: Department of Geography, University of Guelph.

D'Arcy, C., and Siddique, C. M. 1987. Health and unemployment: Findings from a national survey. In *Health and Canadian society* (Second edition), ed. D. Coburn, C. D'Arcy, G. M. Torrance, and P. New, pp. 239–261. Toronto: Fitzhenry and Whiteside.

Davis, K., Gold, M., and Makuc, D. 1981. Access to health care for the poor: Does the gap remain? *Annual Review of Public Health* 2:159–183.

Dear, M. J. 1981. Social and spatial reproduction of the mentally ill. In *Urbanization and urban planning in capitalist society*, ed. M. Dear and A. J. Scott, pp. 481–497. London: Methuen.

Dear, M. J., and Taylor, S.M. 1982. *Not on our street: Community attitudes to mental health*. London: Pion.

Dear, M. J., and Wolch, J. R. 1987. *Landscapes of despair: From deinstitutionalization to homelessness*. Cambridge: Polity.

DeFriese, G. H., and Ricketts, T. C. 1989. Primary health care in rural areas: An agenda for research. *Health Services Research* 23(6):931–973.

Dei Rossi, J. A. n.d. *Physician location choice and state policy: A case study*. Santa Barbara, California: Interplan Corporation.

DeJong, G., and Lifchez, R. 1983. Physical disability and public policy. *Scientific American* 48:240–249.

De la Torre, A., Luft, H., and Fickenscher, K. 1987. *Zips make a difference: Methods to improve identification of rural subgroups*. Draft for Pew Writing Seminar, November 30.

D'Elia, G., and Johnson, I. 1980. Women physicians in a non-metropolitan area. *Journal of Medical Education* 55:580–588.

Denslow, J. S., Hosokawa, M. C., Campbell, J. D., Roberts, C. R., and Samuels, M. E. 1984. Osteopathic physician location and specialty choice. *Journal of Medical Education* 59:655–661.

Deuschle, K. W. 1983. Community oriented primary care: Lessons learned in three decades. In *Community oriented primary care: New directions for health services delivery*, ed. E. Conner and F. Mullan, pp. 1–18. Washington, D.C.: National Academy Press.

Dicker, M., and Sunshine, H. 1988. *Determinants of financially burdensome family health expenses, United States, 1980. National Medical Care Utilization and Expenditure Survey*. Series C, Analytical Report No. 6. Washington, D.C.: National Center for Health Statistics.

Division of National Cost Estimates, Office of the Actuary, Health Care Financing Administration. 1987. Statistical report, National health expenditures, 1986–2000. *Health Care Financing Review* 8(4):1–36.

Doeksen, G. A., Miller, D. A., and Howe, E. 1988. A model to evaluate whether a community can support a physician. *Journal of Medical Education* 63:515–521.

Dohrenwend, B. S., and Dohrenwend, B. P. 1974. *Stressful life events: Their nature and effects*. New York: John Wiley & Sons.

Donovan, P. J., Cline, D. M., Whiltey, T. W., Foster, C., and Outlaw, M. 1989. Prehospital care by EMTs and ENT-Is in a rural setting: Prolongation of scene times by ALS procedures. *Annals of Emergency Medicine* 18:495–500.

Dutton, D. B. 1986. Social class, health and illness. In *Applications of social class in clinical medicine and health policy*, ed. L. Aiken and D. Mechanic, pp. 31–62. New Brunswick, New Jersey: Rutgers University Press.

Eberstein, I. W., and Parker, J. R. 1984. Racial differences in infant mortality by cause of death: The impact of birth weight and maternal age. *Demography* 21(3):309–321.

Elder, G. H., Nguyen, T. V., and Caspi, A. 1985. Linking family hardship to children's lives. *Child Development* 56:361–375.

Elison, G. 1986. Frontier areas: Problems for delivery of health care services. *Rural Health Care* 8(5):1–3.

Elo, I. T., and Beale, C. L. 1988. *The decline in American counter-urbanization in the 1980s.* Paper presented to the Population Association of America, New Orleans, April 21–23.

Emery, R. E. 1982. Interparental conflict and the children of discord and divorce. *Psychological Bulletin* 92:310–330.

Fein, R., and Weber, G. 1971. *Financing medical education: An analysis of alternative policies and mechanisms.* New York: McGraw-Hill.

Feldstein, P. 1983. *Health care economics.* New York: John Wiley & Sons.

Felton, B. J., and Shinn, M. 1981. Ideology and practice of deinstitutionalization. *Journal of Social Issues* 37:158–172.

Ferguson, P. M. 1987. The social construction of mental retardation. *Social Policy* 18:51–56.

Field, N. C. 1986. *Software packages for population analysis on micro-computers with PC or MS DOS. Discussion Paper No. 33.* Toronto: Department of Geography, University of Toronto.

Fine, M., and Asch, A. 1988. Disability beyond stigma: Social interaction, discrimination, and activism. *Journal of Social Issues* 44:3–21.

Fischer, L. R., and Hoffman, C. 1984. Who cares for the elderly: The dilemma of family support. *Research in Social Problems and Public Policy* 3:169–215.

Flinn Foundation. 1989. *Health care in Arizona: A profile.* Phoenix: Flinn Foundation.

Forbes, W. F., Jackson, J. A., and Kraus, A. S. 1987. *Institutionalization of the elderly in Canada.* Toronto: Butterworths.

Forstall, R. 1989. Population Division, Bureau of the Census, U.S. Department of Commerce, Washington, D.C. Personal communication, May 19.

Fort, R. D., and Christianson, J. B. 1981. Determinants of public services provision in rural communities: Evidence from voting on hospital referenda. *Journal of Agricultural Economics* 63:228–235.

Foucault, M. 1989. The politics of health in the eighteenth century. In *Power/knowledge: Selected interviews and other writings 1972–1977*, ed. and trans. C. Gordon, pp. 166–182. Brighton, England: Harvester.

Fournier, G. M., Rasmussen, D. W., and Serow, W. J. 1988. Elderly migration as a response to economic incentives. *Social Science Quarterly* 69:245–260.

Fraser, B. S. 1989. *Service planning for the elderly in rural communities: Learning from the One-Stop Access initiative.* Unpublished M.Sc. thesis, University School of Rural Planning and Development, University of Guelph, Guelph, Ontario, Canada.

Fraser, B. S., and Fuller, A. M. 1989. One-Stop Access for citizens: A model of integrated service delivery for rural areas. In *Aging and health: Linking research and public policy*, ed. S. J. Lewis, pp. 101–110. Chelsea, Michigan: Lewis Publications.

Fraser, B. S., and Martin Matthews, A. 1988. *Simplifying access to services for the elderly in rural areas: How complex a task?* Paper presented to the 17th annual scientific and educational meeting of the Canadian Association on Gerontology, Halifax, Nova Scotia, Canada.

Freeman, H. E., et al. 1987. Americans report on their access to health care. *Health Affairs* 6–17.

Freudenberger, H. 1974. Staff burn-out. *Journal of Social Issues* 30:159–165.

Fruen, M. A., and Cantwell, J. R. 1982. Geographic distribution of physicians: Past trends and future influences. *Inquiry* 19:44–50.

Furman, W., and Buhrmeister, D. 1985. Children's perceptions of the personal relationships in their social networks. *Developmental Psychology* 21:1016–1024.

Garbarino, J., and Crouter, A. 1978. Defining the community context for parent-child relations: The correlates of child maltreatment. *Child Development* 49:604–616.

Garnick, D. W., Luft, H. S., Robinson, J. C., and Tetreault, J. 1987. Appropriate measures of hospital market areas. *Health Services Research* 22(1): 69–90.

Garrison, H. G., Benson, N. H., and Whitley, T. W. 1989. Helicopter use by rural emergency departments to transfer trauma victims: A study of time-to-request intervals. *American Journal of Emergency Medicine* 7(4): 384–386.

Gerontology Research Centre and University School of Rural Planning and Development. 1988. *A proposed model for one-stop access in Huron County, Ontario.* Study prepared for the Huron County Board of Health. Guelph, Ontario, Canada: Gerontology Research Centre and University School of Rural Planning and Development, University of Guelph.

Geyman, J. P., Cherkin, D. C., Deisher, J. B., and Gordon, M. J. 1980. Graduate follow-up in the University of Washington Family Practice Residency network. *Journal of Family Practice* 11(5):743–752.

Gibbens, B. P., and Ludtke, R. L. 1989. *Rural hospital conversion: State action.* Grand Forks, North Dakota: University of North Dakota Rural Health Research Center.

Gilford, D. M., Nelson, G. L., and Ingram, L. 1981. *Rural America in Passage: Statistics for Policy.* Washington, D.C.: National Academy Press.

Gilligan, T., Mitchell, S. A., and Scott, J. 1988. Special report: Rural hospitals—The crisis is now. *Federation of American Health Systems Review* 21(6):27–28, 33.

Gish, O. 1971. *Doctor migration and world health.* Occasional Papers on Social Administration, No. 43, Social Administration Research Trust. London: G. Bell and Sons.

Gjerde, C., and Parker, L. 1983. Practice selection factors: A follow-up of 74 graduates of an Iowa residency program. *Family Medicine* 15(3):83–87.

Glaser, M., Sarnowski, A. A., and Sheth, B. 1982. Career choices from medical school to practice: Findings from a regional clinical education site. *Journal of Medical Education* 57:442–448.

Gordon, R. J. 1987. *The Arizona rural health provider atlas,* Second Edition. Tucson: Rural Health Office, University of Arizona.

Gordon, R. J., and Higgins, B. A. 1991. *Declining availability of rural physician obstetric service and medical malpractice.* Paper presented to the annual meeting of the Association of American Geographers, Miami, Florida, April 15.

Gordon, R. J., McMullen, G., Weiss, B. D., and Nichols, A. W. 1987. The effect of malpractice liability on the delivery of rural obstetrical care. *Journal of Rural Health* 3(1):7–13.

Goudy, W. J., and Dobson, C. 1988. Work, retirement, and financial situations of the rural elderly. In *The elderly in rural society,* ed. R. T. Coward and G. R. Lee. New York: Springer-Verlag.

Graham, R. 1988. *Building community support for people: A plan for mental health in Ontario.* Toronto: Ministry of Health.

Gray, P. G., and Cartwright, A. 1953. Choosing and changing doctors. *Lancet* 2:1308–1309.

Greenberg, M. R. 1983. *Urbanization and cancer mortality.* New York: Oxford University Press.

———. 1987a. The changing geography of major causes of death among middle age white Americans, 1938–1981. *Socio-Economic Planning Science* 21(4):223–228.

———. 1987b. Urban/rural differences in behavioral risk factors for chronic diseases. *Urban Geography* 8(2):146–151.

Greenberg, M., Barrows, D., Clark, P., Grohs, S., Kaplan, S., and Newton, N. 1983. White female respiratory cancer mortality: A geographical anomaly. *Lung* 161:235–243.

Greenberg, M. R., Carey, G. W., and Popper, F. J. 1985. External causes of death among young white Americans. *New England Journal of Medicine* 313(23):1483.

Grescoe, P. 1987. A nation's disgrace. In *Health and Canadian society* (Second edition), ed. D. Coburn, C. D'Arcy, G. M. Torrance, and P. New, pp. 127–140. Toronto: Fitzhenry and Whiteside.

Gross, J. M., and Schwenger, C. W. 1981. *Health care costs for the elderly in Ontario: 1976–2026.* Occasional Paper No. 11. Toronto: Ontario Economic Council.

Grundy, E. 1987. Retirement migration and its consequences in England and Wales. *Ageing and Society* 7: 57–82.

Gurney, R. M. 1980. The effects of unemployment on the psycho-social development of school leavers. *Journal of Occupational Psychology* 53: 205–213.

Guterman, S., Eggers, P., Riley, G., Greene T., and Terrell S. 1988. The first 3 years of Medicare prospective payment: An overview. *Health Care Financing Review* 9(3):67–77.

Alan Guttmacher Institute. 1989. *Prenatal care in the United States: A state and county inventory.* New York: Alan Guttmacher Institute.

Haber, L., and McNeil, J. 1983. *Methodological questions in the estimation of disability prevalence.* Washington, D.C.: Population Division, U.S. Bureau of the Census.

Hadley, J. 1988. Medicare spending and mortality rates of the elderly. *Inquiry* 25:485–493.

Hafferty, F. W. 1986. Physician oversupply as a socially constructed reality. *Journal of Health and Social Behavior* 27(4):358–369.

Haggett, P. 1965. *Locational analysis in human geography.* London: Edward Arnold.

Hahn, H. 1988. The politics of physical differences: Disability and discrimination. *Journal of Social Issues* 44:39–47.

———. 1989. Disability and the reproduction of bodily images: The dynamics of human appearances. In *The power of geography*, ed. M. Dear and J. Wolch, pp. 370–388. Boston: Unwin Hyman.

Hale, F. A., McConnochie, K. M., Chapman, R. J., and Whiting, R. D. 1979. The impact of a required preceptorship on senior medical students. *Journal of Medical Education* 54:396–401.

Hall, G. B., Roseman, C. R., and Joseph, A. E. 1986. The changing geography of the elderly in metropolitan Auckland: Pattern, process and policy implications. *New Zealand Geographer* 42:46–56.

Hare, P. H., and Hollis, L. E. 1983. Saving the suburbs for schoolchildren. *Journal of Housing for the Elderly* 7:69–79.

Hargrove, D. 1982. An overview of professional considerations in the rural community. In *Handbook of rural community mental health*, ed. P. Kellar and J. Murray, pp. 169–182. New York: Human Sciences Press.

Harris, D. L., Coleman, M., and Mallea, M. 1982. Impact of participation in a family practice tract program on student career decisions. *Journal of Medical Education* 57:609–614.

Hart, L. G., Rosenblatt, R. A., and Amundson, B. A. 1989. *Rural hospital utilization: Who stays and who goes?* Rural Health Working Paper Series, Vol. 1, No. 2. Seattle: WAMI Rural Health Research Center, Department of Family Medicine, University of Washington.

Hassinger, E. W., Gill, L. S., Hageman, R., and Hobbs, D. J. 1979. *A restudy of rural physicians in twenty rural Missouri counties.* DHEW Publication No. (HRA) 79-634. Hyattsville, Maryland: Office of Graduate Medical Education, Health Resources Administration, U.S. Department of Health, Education, and Welfare.

Hawes, J. M., and Lumpkin, J. R. 1984. Understanding the outshopper. *Journal of the Academy of Marketing Science* 12:200–218.

Hawkins, M. L. 1988. The trauma score: A simple method to evaluate quality of care. *American Surgeon* 54(4):204–206.

Health and activity limitation survey 1986. Ottawa: Statistics Canada.

Health and Welfare Canada. 1983. *Fact book on aging in Canada.* Ottawa: Minister of National Health and Welfare.

————. 1989. *Charting Canada's future: A report of the demographic review.* Ottawa: Minister of National Health and Welfare.

Health Economics Research. 1988. *New Jersey MICU Evaluation Project.* Needham, Massachusetts: Health Economics Research, Inc.

Hecht, R. C., and Farrell, J. G. 1982. Graduate follow-up in the University of Wisconsin Family Practice Residency program. *Journal of Family Practice* 14(3):549–555.

Hedges, J. R., Feero, S., Moore, B., Haver, D. W., and Shultz, B. 1987. Comparison of prehospital trauma triage instruments in a semirural population. *Journal of Emergency Medicine* 5(3):197–208.

Held, P. J. 1973. *The migration of the 1955–65 graduates of American medical schools.* Berkeley, California: Ford Foundation Research Program in University Administration.

Hendricks, A. 1989. *Hospital closures have little effect on reducing bed capacity.* Research Update. Needham, Massachussets: Health Economics Research, Inc., and Center for Health Economics Research.

Hersh, A. S., and Van Hook, R. T. 1989. A research agenda for rural health services. *Health Services Research* 23(6):1053–1064.

Heseltine, G. F. 1983. *Towards a blueprint for change: A mental health policy and program perspective.* Toronto: Ministry of Health.

Hewitt, M. 1989. *Defining rural areas: Impact on health care policy and research.* Office of Technology Assessment Staff Paper. Washington, D.C.: U.S. Government Printing Office.

Hodge, G. 1987. *The elderly in Canada's small towns: Recent trends and their implications.* Occasional Paper No. 43. Vancouver, British Columbia, Canada: Centre for Human Settlement, University of British Columbia.

Hogan, C. 1988. Patterns of travel for rural individuals hospitalized in New York State: Relationships between distance, destination and case mix. *Journal of Rural Health* 4:29–41.

Holmes, J. E., and Miller, D. A. 1986. Factors affecting decisions on practice locations. *Journal of Medical Education* 61:721–726.

Holt, T. 1989. I cannot afford to go to medical school. *New England Journal of Medicine* 320(24):1630.

Hook, N. 1991. Regional Administrator, Clinica Adelnorté Inc., El Mirage, Arizona. Personal interview, August 7.

Horner, R. D. 1988. Impact of federal primary health care policy in rural areas: Empirical evidence from the literature. *Journal of Rural Health* 4(2):13–28.

Hough, D. E., and Marder, W. D. 1982. State retention of medical school graduates. *Journal of Medical Education* 57:505–526.

Houtchens, B. 1977. Initial evaluation and management of major trauma in the rural setting: An appeal for a national standard. *Legal Aspects of Medical Practice* 5(12):38–39.

Hymel, S., and Rubin, K. H. 1985. Children with peer relationship and social skills problems: Conceptual, methodological, and developmental issues. In *Annals of child development*, Vol. 2, ed. G. I. Whitehurst, pp. 251–297. Greenwich, Connecticut: JAI Press.

Hynes, K., and Givner, N. 1983. Physician distribution in a predominantly rural state: Predictors and trends. *Inquiry* 20:185–190.

Ison, T. G. 1983. *Workers' compensation in Canada.* Toronto: Butterworths.

Robert Wood Johnson Foundation. 1978. *Special report. A new survey on access to medical care.* No. 1. Princeton, New Jersey: Robert Wood Johnson Foundation.

———. 1983. *Special report. Updated report on access to health care for the American people.* No. 1. Princeton, New Jersey: Robert Wood Johnson Foundation.

———. 1987. *Special report. Access to health care in the United States: Results of a 1986 survey.* No. 2. Princeton, New Jersey: Robert Wood Johnson Foundation.

Johnston, P. 1983. *Native children and the child welfare system.* Toronto: Canadian Council on Social Development.

Jonas, S. 1986. Health manpower. In *Health care delivery in the United States,* ed. S. Jonas, pp. 54–89. New York: Springer-Verlag.

Joseph, A. E., and Bantock, P. R. 1984. Rural accessibility of general practitioners: The case of Bruce and Grey Counties, Ontario, 1901–1981. *Canadian Geographer* 28:226–239.

Joseph, A. E., and Cloutier, D. S. 1989. Elderly migration and its implications for health service provision in rural communities: An Ontario perspective. Paper presented to a conference on Geographical Perspectives on Health and Ageing, Institute of Human Ageing, University of Liverpool, Liverpool, England.

———. 1990. A framework for modeling the consumption of health services by the rural elderly. *Social Science and Medicine* 30:45–52.

Joseph, A. E., and Fuller, A. M. 1991. Towards an integrative perspective on the housing, services and transportation implications of rural aging. *Canadian Journal on Aging* 10:127–148.

Joseph, A. E., and Phillips, D. R. 1984. *Accessibility and utilization: Geographical perspectives on health care delivery.* London: Harper & Row.

Joseph, A. E., Keddie, P. D., and Smit, B. E. 1988. Unravelling the population turnaround in rural Canada. *Canadian Geographer* 32:17–30.

Kane, R. L. 1969. Determination of health care priorities and expectations among rural consumers. *Health Services Research* 4:142–151.

Kane, R. L., Warnick, R., Proctor, P., Olsen, D. M., and Gourley, D. 1975. Mail-order medicine: An analysis of the Sears Roebuck Foundation's community medical assistance program. *Journal of the American Medical Association* 232:1023–1027.

Kasteler, J., Kane, R. L., Olsen, D. M., and Thetford, C. 1976. Issues underlying prevalence of "doctor shopping" behavior. *Journal of Health and Social Behavior* 17:328–339.

Kaufman, A., Satcher, D., Jackson, R., Lewis, M., and Duban, S. 1983. Undergraduate education for rural, primary care: Strategies for institutional change at New Mexico and Morehouse. *Family Medicine* 15(1):20–24.

Kennedy, V. C., Linder, S. H., and Spears, W. D. 1987. Estimating the impact of state manpower policy: A case study of reducing medical school enrollments. *Journal of Health Politics, Policy and Law* 12(2):299–311.

Kindig, D. A., and Movassaghi, H. 1987. *Trends in physician supply and characteristics in small rural counties of the United States 1975–1985.* Kansas City, Missouri: National Rural Health Association.

———. 1989. The adequacy of physician supply in small rural counties. *Health Affairs* 8(2):63–76.

Koska, M. T. 1988. FMG residents expensive to replace. *Hospitals* 62(10):77.

Kramer, M. 1980. The rising pandemic of mental disorders and associated chronic diseases and disabilities. In *Epidemiological research as basis for the organization of extramural psychiatry,* ed. E. Strömgren, A. Dupont, and J. A. Nielsen, pp. 382–397. *Acta Psychiatrica Scandinavica* 62 (suppl. 285).

Krob, M. J., Cram, A. E., Vargish, T., et al. 1984. Rural trauma care: A study of trauma care in a rural emergency medical services region. *Annals of Emergency Medicine* 13:891–895.

Krout, J. 1988. The elderly in rural environments. *Journal of Rural Studies* 4:103–114.

Lakin, K. C., and Bruininks, R. H. 1985. Contemporary services for handicapped children and youth. In *Living and learning in the least restrictive environment,* ed. R. H. Bruininks and K. C. Lakin, pp. 3–22. Baltimore: Paul H. Brookes.

Landau, T. P., Ledley, R. S., Champion, H. R., and Sacco, W. J. 1982. Decision theory model of the emergency triage process. *Computers in Biology and Medicine* 12(1):27–42.

Langwell, K., Nelson, S., Calvin, D., and Drabek, J. 1985. Characteristics of rural communities and the changing geographic distribution of physicians. *Journal of Rural Health* 1(2):42–55.

Langwell, K., Drabek, J., Nelson, S. L., and Lenk, E. 1987. Effects of community characteristics on young physicians' decisions regarding rural practice. *Public Health Reports* 102(3):317–328.

Larson, D. M., and Mellstrom, M. S. 1987. Management of multiple trauma in a rural setting. *Minnesota Medicine* 70(1):43–45.

Lassey, W. R. 1977. *Planning in rural environments.* New York: McGraw-Hill.

Lazenby, H. C., and Letsch, S. W. 1990. National health expenditures, 1989. *Health Care Financing Review* 12(2):1–26.

Lee, A. S. 1980. Impact of aging on service delivery. *Research on Aging* 2:243–253.

Lee, P., LeRoy, L., Stalcup, J., and Beck, J. 1976. *Primary care in a specialized world.* Cambridge, Massachussets: Ballinger.

Leicht, M. J., Dula, D. J., Brotman, S., Anderson, T. E., Gesner, H. W., Parrish, G. A., and Rose, W. D. 1986. Rural interhospital helicopter transport of motor vehicle trauma victims: Causes for delays and recommendations. *Annals of Emergency Medicine* 15(4):450–453.

Lempers, J. D., Clark-Lempers, D., and Simons, R. L. 1989. Economic hardship, parenting, and distress in adolescence. *Child Development* 60:25–39.

Leonardson, G., Lapierre, R., and Hollingsworth, D. 1985. Factors predictive of physician location. *Journal of Medical Education* 60:37–43.

Lewis, D. L. 1985. *Special purpose passenger transport: The economics of serving the travel needs of handicapped persons.* Unpublished Ph.D. thesis, Department of Geography, University of London.

Ley, D. 1985. Cultural/humanistic geography. *Progress in Human Geography* 9:415–423.

Licht, H. 1989. Program Manager, Primary Care Section, Public Health Division, New Mexico State Health and Environment Department, Santa Fe, New Mexico. Personal communication, May.

Lichter, D. T., Fuguitt, G. V., and Heaton, T. B. 1985. Components of nonmetropolitan population change: The contributions of rural areas. *Rural Sociology* 50(1):88–98.

Lichter, D. T., Henton, T. B., and Fuguitt, G. V. 1986. Convergence in black and white population redistribution in the U.S. *Social Science Quarterly* 67(1):21–38.

Lithwick, N. H., Schiff, M., and Vernon, E. 1986. *An overview of registered Indian conditions in Canada.* Ottawa: Ministry of Indian and Northern Affairs.

Little, D. L. 1980. Changing demographic patterns and some potential implications for nonmetropolitan America. In *Special Study on Economic Change,* Vol. 1: *Human resources and demographics: Characteristics of people and policy.* Joint Economic Committee, Congress of the United States, pp. 153–168. Washington, D.C.: U.S. Government Printing Office.

Lomas, J., Stoddart, G. L., and Barer, M. L. 1985. Supply projections as planning: A critical review of forecasting net physician requirements in Canada. *Social Science and Medicine* 20(4):411–424.

Long, E. 1975. *The geographic distribution of physicians in the U.S.: An evaluation of policy related research.* Report prepared for the National Science Foundation, NSF-C814. Minneapolis, Minnesota: Interstudy.

Long, L., and DeAre, D. 1982. Repopulating the countryside: A 1980 census trend. *Science* 217:1111–1116.

Longino, C. F., and Biggar, J. C. 1982. The impact of population redistribution on service delivery. *Gerontologist* 22:153–159.

Lorber, J. 1984. *Women physicians*. New York: Tavistock Press.

Ludtke, R. L., Geller, J. M., Hart, J. P., and Fickenscher, K. M. 1989. *Relationships between site, access variables and loss of local clientele*. Paper presented to the 12th annual meeting of the National Rural Health Association, Reno, Nevada, May 1.

McCarthy, K. F. 1983. *The elderly population's changing spatial distribution. Patterns of change since 1960*. Santa Monica, California: Rand Corporation.

McConnell, C. E., and Tobias, L. A. 1986. Distributional change in physician manpower, United States, 1963–80. *American Journal of Public Health* 76:638–642.

McDaniel, S. 1986. *Canada's aging population*. Toronto: Butterworths.

McEniry, M. 1988. *Report of the Arizona Health Education Centers program*. Tucson, Arizona: Rural Health Office, University of Arizona College of Medicine.

McGranahan, D. A., Hession, J. C., Hines, F. K., and Jordan, M. F. 1986. *Social and economic characteristics of the population in metro and nonmetro counties, 1970–80*. Economic Research Service, U.S. Department of Agriculture, Rural Development Research Report No. 58. Washington, D.C.: U.S. Government Printing Office.

McGuirk, M. A., and Porrell, F. W. 1984. Spatial patterns of hospital utilization: The impact of distance and time. *Inquiry* 21:84–95.

McKay, S. 1987. Social work in Canada's north: Survival and development issues affecting aboriginal and industry-based communities. *International Social Work* 30:259–278.

McKenzie, B. Y., and LaMacchia, R. A. 1987. *The U.S. Geological Survey–U.S. Bureau of the Census Cooperative Digital Mapping Project: A unique success story*. Washington, D.C.: U.S. Government Printing Office.

McLaughlin, C. P., Ricketts, T. C., Freund, D. A., and Sheps, C. G. 1985. An evaluation of subsidized rural primary care programs. IV. Impact of the rural hospital on clinic self-sufficiency. *American Journal of Public Health*. 75:749–753.

McShane, D. 1987. Mental health and North American Indian/Native communities: Cultural transactions, education, and regulation. *American Journal of Community Psychology* 15:95–116.

MacStravic, R. S. 1987. Loyalty of hospital patients: A vital marketing objective. *Health Care Management Review* 12:23–30.

Madison, D. L. 1980. Managing a chronic problem: The rural physician shortage. *Annals of Internal Medicine* 92:852–854.

Magnusson, G. 1980. The role of proximity in the use of hospital emergency departments. *Sociology of Health and Illness* 2:203–214.

Maheux, B., Pineault, R., Lambert, J., Beland, F., and Levesque, A. 1990. Primary care in Quebec: A comparison between private practitioners and physicians working in public community health centers. *Canadian Journal of Public Health* 81(1):27–31.

Manard, B. B., and Lewin, L. S. 1983. *Physician supply and distribution: Issues and options for state policy makers*. Washington, D.C.: National Center for Health Services Research, Office of the Assistant Secretary for Health, U.S. Department of Health and Human Services.

Manga, P. 1987. Equality of access and inequalities in health status: Policy implications of a paradox. In *Health and Canadian society* (Second edition), ed. D. Coburn, C. D'Arcy, G. M. Torrance, and P. New, pp. 637–648. Toronto: Fitzhenry and Whiteside.

Manning, W. G., Newhouse, J. P., Daun, N., Keeler, E. B., Benjamin, B., Liebowitz, A., Marquis, M. S., and Zwanziger, J. 1988. *Health insurance and the demand for medical care. Evidence from a randomized experiment.* Rand Health Insurance Experiment Series. Santa Monica, California: Rand Corporation.

Manton, K. G., and Soldo, B. J. 1985. Dynamics of health changes in the oldest old: New perspectives and evidence. *Milbank Memorial Fund Quarterly* 63(2):206–285.

Manton, K. G., and Stallard, E. 1982. Temporal trends in U.S. multiple cause of death mortality data: 1968–1977. *Demography* 19(4):527–547.

Mantovani, R. E., Gordon, T. L., and Johnson, P. G. 1976. *Medical student indebtedness and career plans, 1974–1975.* DHEW (HRA) 77-21. Washington, D.C.: U.S. Government Printing Office.

Marder, W. D. 1974. Practice patterns of new community-based medical schools. *Journal of Medical Education* 59:345–346.

Martin Matthews, A. 1988. Variations in the conceptualization and measurement of rurality: Conflicting findings on the elderly widowed. *Journal of Rural Studies* 4:141–150.

Martin Matthews, A., and Vanden Heuvel, A. 1987. Conceptual and methodological issues in research on aging in rural versus urban environments. *Canadian Journal on Aging* 5:49–60.

Martin, L. F., Richardson, J. D., Bell, R. A., and Polk, H. C. 1971. The initial impact of a surgical AHES program on medical students' career decisions. *Journal of Medical Education* 56:812–817.

Massam, B. H., and Askew, I. 1984. A theoretical perspective on rural service provision: A systems approach. In *Rural public services: International comparisons*, ed. R. E. Lonsdale and G. Enyedi, pp. 15–38. Boulder, Colorado: Westview.

Mattson, D. E., Stehr, D. C., and Will, R. E. 1973. Evaluation of a program designed to produce rural physicians. *Journal of Medical Education* 48:323–331.

Mayer, E. S. 1988. *Progress report of the North Carolina Area Health Education Centers (AHEC) program.* Chapel Hill, North Carolina: University of North Carolina at Chapel Hill School of Medicine.

Mayer, J. D. 1983. The distance behavior of hospital patients: A disaggregated analysis. *Social Science and Medicine* 17(12):819–827.

Mayer, J. D., Kohlenberg, E. R., Sieferman, G. E., and Rosenblatt, R. A. 1987. Patterns of rural hospital closure in the United States. *Social Science and Medicine* 24:327–334.

Meade, M. S., Florin, J. W., and Gesler, W. M. 1988. Health care resources. In *Medical geography*, ed. M. S. Meade et al., pp. 282–305. New York: Guilford Press.

Melcher, J. 1988. *The rural health care challenge.* Staff Report to the Special Committee on Aging, United States Senate. Washington, D.C.: U.S. Government Printing Office.

Merlis, M. 1989. *Rural Hospitals.* Congressional Research Service Report for Congress. Washington, D.C.: Library of Congress.

Mick, S. S., and Worobey, J. L. 1986. The future role of foreign medical graduates in U. S. medical practice: Projections into the 1990's. *Health Services Research* 21(1):85–106.

Miller, C. A., Moos, M., Kotch, J., Brown, M. L., and Brainard, M. P. 1981. Role of health departments in the delivery of ambulatory care. *American Journal of Public Health* 71(suppl.):15–29.

Minister for Senior Citizens' Affairs. 1986. *A new agenda: Health and social service strategies for Ontario's seniors*. Toronto: Office for Senior Citizens' Affairs.

Ministry of Community and Social Services of Ontario. 1980. *Consultation paper: Children's services past, present and future*. Toronto: Government of Ontario.

Ministry of Community and Social Services, North Region. 1988. *Northern directions for the delivery of services to special needs children and their families*. Toronto: Government of Ontario.

Ministry of Mines and Northern Development. 1986. *Final report and recommendations of the advisory committee on resource dependent communities in northern Ontario*. Toronto: Government of Ontario.

Ministry of Municipal Affairs. 1986. *Planned retirement communities*. Toronto: Ministry of Municipal Affairs.

Missouri Health Facilities Review Committee. 1989. Missouri air ambulance report. Jefferson City, Missouri: The Missouri Certificate of Need Program.

Moore, E. G., Burke, S. O., and Rosenberg, M. W. 1989. *An atlas of the elderly population of Canada*. Kingston, Ontario, Canada: Department of Geography, Queen's University.

Morrill, R. L. 1988. Migration regions and population redistribution. *Growth and Change* 19:43–60.

Morrisey, M. A., Sloan, F. A., and Valvona, J. 1989. Defining geographic markets for hospital care. *Law and Contemporary Problems* 51:165–194.

Moscovice, I. 1989. Rural hospitals: A literature synthesis and health services research agenda. *Health Services Research* 23:891–930.

Moscovice, I., and Rosenblatt, R. 1982a. Rural health care delivery amidst federal retrenchment: Lessons from the Robert Wood Johnson Foundation's rural practice project. *American Journal of Public Health* 72(12): 1380–1385.

———. 1982b. *The viability of the rural hospital*. Hyattsville, Maryland: National Center for Health Services Research.

———. 1985. A prognosis for the rural hospital, Part I: What is the role of the rural hospital? *Journal of Rural Health* 1(1):29–40.

———. 1985. A prognosis for the rural hospital, Part II: Are rural hospitals economically viable? *Journal of Rural Health* 1(2):11–33.

Moseley, M. J. 1979. *Accessibility: The rural challenge*. London: Methuen.

Mueller, B. A., Rivara, F. P., and Bergman, A. B. 1988. Urban-rural location and the risk of dying in a pedestrian-vehicle collision. *Journal of Trauma* 28(1):91–94.

Mullner, R. M., and McNeil, D. 1986. Rural and urban hospital closures: A comparison. *Health Affairs* 5:131–141.

Mullner, R. M., Rydman, R. J., Whiteis, D. G., and Rich, R. F. 1988. *Rural community hospital closure in the United States: An epidemiologic matched case-control study*. Unpublished paper. Chicago: Center for

Health Services Research, School of Public Health, University of Illinois at Chicago.

———. 1989. Rural community hospitals and factors correlated with their risk of closing. *Public Health Reports* 104:315–325.

Murrin, K. L. 1982. Laying the groundwork: Issues facing rural primary care. In *Management of rural primary care: Concepts and cases,* ed. G. E. Bisbee, Jr. Chicago: Hospital Research and Educational Trust.

National Academy of Sciences. 1966. Accidental death and disability— The neglected disease of modern society. Washington, D.C.: National Academy Press.

National Advisory Council on Aging. 1986. *Toward a community support policy for Canadians.* Ottawa: Government of Canada.

National Association of Community Health Centers and National Rural Health Association. 1988. *Health care in rural America: The crisis unfolds.* Report to the Joint Task Force of the National Association of Community Health Centers and the National Rural Health Association.

National Coalition for Agricultural Safety and Health. 1988. *Agriculture at risk—A report to the nation. Agricultural occupational and environmental health: Policy strategies for the future,* ed. J. A. Merchant, B. C. Kross, K. J. Donham, and D. S. Pratt. Iowa City, Iowa: Institute of Agricultural Medicine and Occupational Health.

National Rural Electric Cooperative Association. 1988a. *Survey of health coverage in smaller firms: Evidence and policy implications,* June. Washington, D.C.: National Rural Electric Cooperative Association.

———. 1988b. *Minimum health benefit: A comparison of provisions and costs,* July. Washington, D.C.: National Rural Electric Cooperative Association.

National Rural Health Association. 1988a. NRHA files lawsuit against HHS. *Rural Health Care* 10(6):1–2.

———. 1988b. *Community health centers and the rural economy: The struggle for survival.* Kansas City, Missouri: National Rural Health Association and National Association of Community Health Centers.

———. 1989. House Rural Health Care Coalition sets goals. *Rural Health Care* 11(1):7.

Naylor, C. D. 1986. *Private practice, Canadian medicine and the politics of health insurance 1911–1966.* Montreal: McGill-Queen's University Press.

Nelson, L., Ciemnecki, A., Carlton, N., and Langwell, K. 1989. *Assignment and the participating physician program: An analysis of beneficiary awareness, understanding, and experience.* Background Paper No. 89-1. Prepared for the Physician Payment Review Commission. Washington, D.C.: Physician Payment Review Commission.

New Mexico State Health and Environment Department. 1987. *Frontier areas in New Mexico—1987.* Unpublished concept paper. Santa Fe, New Mexico: Public Health Division, Primary Care Section, New Mexico State Health and Environment Department.

New York State Commission on Graduate Medical Education. 1986. *Report of the New York State Commission on Graduate Medical Education.* Albany, New York: New York State Commission on Graduate Medical Education.

New York Times. 1986. Census study reports one in five adults suffers from disability. December 23: 67.

———. 1989. As farms falter, rural homelessness grows. May 2: A1, C2.

Newhouse, J. P.. 1982. *The geographic distribution of physicians. Is the conventional wisdom correct?* Santa Monica, California: Rand Corporation.

Newhouse, J. P., Williams, A. P., Bennett, B. W., and Schwartz, W. B. 1982a. Where have all the doctors gone? *Journal of the American Medical Association* 247(17):2392–2396.

———. 1982b. *How have location patterns of physicians affected the availability of medical services?* Santa Monica, California: Rand Corporation.

Neysmith, S. 1988. Canadian social services and social work practice in the field of aging. *Journal of Gerontological Social Work* 12:41–60.

Northcott, H. 1980. Convergence or divergence: The rural-urban distribution of physicians and dentists in census divisions and incorporated cities, towns, and villages in Alberta, Canada, 1956–1976. *Social Science and Medicine* 41D:17–22.

———. 1988. *Changing residence: The geographic mobility of elderly Canadians.* Toronto: Butterworths.

Norton, C. H., and McManus, M. A. 1989. Background tables on demographic characteristics, health status and health services utilization. *Health Services Research* 23(6):725–757.

Office of Technology Assessment, U.S. Congress. 1986. *Payment for physician services: Strategies for Medicare.* Washington, D.C.: U.S. Government Printing Office.

———. 1989. *Special report: Rural emergency services.* Washington, D.C.: U.S. Government Printing Office.

Offord, D. R., Boyle, M. H., Szatmari, P., Rae-Grant, N., Links, P. S., Cadman, D. T., Byles, J. A., Crawford, J. W., Blum, H. M., Byrne, C., Thomas, H., and Woodward, C. A. 1987. Ontario child health study: II. Six-month prevalence of disorder and rates of service utilization. *Archives of General Psychiatry* 44:832–836.

Olmsted, F. L. [1970.] *Public parks and the enlightenment of towns.* New York: Arno Press.

O'Hare, W. P. 1988. *The rise of poverty in rural america.* Population Trends and Public Policy Series, No. 15. Washington, D.C.: Population Reference Bureau.

O'Neil, J. D. 1987. Health care in a central Canadian Arctic community. In *Health and Canadian society* (Second edition), ed. D. Coburn, C. D'Arcy, G. M. Torrance, and P. New, pp. 141–158. Toronto: Fitzhenry and Whiteside.

Ontario Advisory Council on Senior Citizens. 1980. *Towards an understanding of the rural elderly.* Toronto: Ontario Advisory Council on Senior Citizens.

Ornoto, J. P., Craven, E. J., and Nelson, N. M. 1985. Impact of improved emergency medical services and emergency trauma care on the reduction in mortality from trauma. *Journal of Trauma* 25(7):575–579.

Paine, W., ed. 1982. *Job stress and burnout: Research, theory, and intervention perspectives.* Beverly Hills, California: Sage.

Paiva, R. E. A., Vu, N. V., and Verhulst, S. J. 1982. The effect of clinical experiences in medical school on specialty choice decisions. *Journal of Medical Education* 57:666–674.

Palsbo, S. J. 1989. *The AAPCC explained.* Research Brief No. 8. Washington, D. C.: Group Health Association of America.

Parker, J. G., and Asher, S. R. 1987. Peer relations and later personal adjustment: Are low-accepted children at risk? *Psychological Bulletin* 102:357–389.

Parker, R. C., and Sorensen, A. A. 1978. The tides of rural physicians. The ebb and flow, or why physicians move out of and into small communities. *Medical Care* 16(2):152–166.

Parliamentary Committee on Equality of Rights. 1985. *"Equality for all." The report of the parliamentary committee on equality rights.* Ottawa: Supply and Services Canada.

Patrick, D. L. 1989. A socio-medical approach to disablement. In *Disablement in the community*, ed. D. L. Patrick and H. Peach, pp. 1–18. Oxford: Oxford University Press.

Patterson, E. P., II. 1972. *The Canadian Indian: A history since 1500.* Toronto: Collier Macmillan Canada.

Patterson, G. R., DeBaryshe, B. D., and Ramsey, E. 1989. A developmental perspective on antisocial behaviour. *American Psychologist* 44:329–335.

Patton, L. 1989. Setting the rural health services research agenda: The Congressional perspective. *Health Services Research* 23(6):1005–1052.

Physician Payment Review Commission. 1988. *Annual report to Congress.* Washington, D.C.: Physician Payment Review Commission.

Pickard, J. 1988. A new county classification system. *Appalachia* 21(3):19–24.

Politzer, R. M., Morrow, J. S., and Sudia, R. K. 1978. Foreign-trained physicians in American medicine: A case study. *Medical Care* 16(8):611–627.

Pollard, J. H. 1988. On the decomposition of changes in expectation of life and differentials in life expectancy. *Demography* 25(2):265–276.

Popper, F. J. 1986. The strange case of the contemporary American frontier. *Yale Review* 76(1):101–121.

Pred, A. R. 1966. *The spatial dynamics of U.S. urban-industrial growth, 1800–1914.* Cambridge, Massachussets: MIT Press.

Prospective Payment Assessment Commission. 1988. *An evaluation of the Department of Health and Human Services' report to Congress on studies of urban-rural and related geographical adjustments in the Medicare Prospective Payment System.* Washington, D.C.: U.S. Government Printing Office.

———. 1989. *Report and recommendations to the Secretary* [U.S. Department of Health and Human Services]. Washington, D.C.: U.S. Government Printing Office.

Pust, R. E., and Moher, L. M. 1983. Promoting medical careers in underserved areas: The C.U.P. program at the University of Arizona. *Arizona Medicine* 40:397–401.

Rabinowitz, H. K. 1983. A program to recruit and educate medical students to practice family medicine in underserved areas. *Journal of the American Medical Association* 249(8):1038–1041.

———. 1988. Evaluation of a selective medical school admissions policy to increase the number of family physicians in rural and underserved areas. *New England Journal of Medicine* 319(8):480–486.

Richichi, E. 1988. *Immigration, health status, and utilization of medical services: The case of Mexican-Americans.* Unpublished Ph.D. dissertation. Department of Health Policy and Administration, University of North Carolina at Chapel Hill.

Ricketts, T. C., Guild, P. A., Sheps, C. G., and Wagner, E. H. 1984. An evaluation of subsidized rural primary care programs: III. Stress and survival, 1981–82. *American Journal of Public Health* 74(8):816–819.

Roemer, M. I. 1948. Historic development of the current crisis of rural medicine in the United States. In *Victor Robinson memorial volume: Essays in history of medicine*, ed. S. Kagan, pp. 333–342. New York: Froeben Press.

Rogers, A., and Woodward, J. 1988. The sources of regional elderly population growth: Migration and aging-in-place. *Professional Geographer* 40:450–458.

Roghmann, K. H., and Zastowny, S. R. 1979. Proximity as a factor in the selection of health care providers: Emergency room visits compared to obstetric admissions and abortions. *Social Science and Medicine* 13:61–69.

Roos, N. P. 1989. How a universal health care system responds to an aging population. *Journal of Aging and Health* 1:411–429.

Rosenberg, M. W. 1983. Accessibility to health care: A North American perspective. *Progress in Human Geography* 7:78–87.

Rosenberg, M. W., Moore, E. G., and Ball, S. 1989. Components of change in the spatial distribution of the elderly population in Ontario, 1976–86. *Canadian Geographer* 33:218–229.

Rosenberg, S. 1988. Rural Health Clinics Act certification benefits. *Rural Health Care* 10(3):7.

Rosenblatt, R. A. 1981. Health and health services. In *Nonmetropolitan America in transition*, ed. A. H. Hawley and S. M. Mazie, pp. 614–642. Chapel Hill, North Carolina: University of North Carolina Press.

Rosenblatt, R. A., and Moscovice, I. 1978. The growth and evaluation of rural primary care practice: The National Health Service Corps experience in the Northwest. *Medical Care* 16(10):819–827.

———. 1979. *The National Health Service Corps program: A review and discussion of past research and evaluation efforts*. Purchase Order No. 298851. Washington, D.C.: Department of Health, Education and Welfare.

———. 1980. The National Health Service Corps: Rapid growth and uncertain future. *Milbank Memorial Fund Quarterly* 58:282–309.

———. 1982. *Rural health care*. New York: John Wiley & Sons.

Rosenwaike, I. 1985. A demographic portrait of the oldest old. *Milbank Memorial Fund Quarterly* 63:187–205.

Ross, P. J. 1986. Remarks on the development of a policy-oriented classification of nonmetropolitan counties. In proceedings of Rural people and places: A symposium on typology, Grantville, Pennsylvania, October 22–24. Washington, D.C.: Economic Research Service, U.S. Department of Agriculture.

Rowland, A. J., and Cooper, P. 1983. *Environment and health*. Baltimore, Maryland: Edward Arnold.

Rowland, D., and Lyons, B. 1989. Triple jeopardy: Rural, poor, and uninsured. *Health Services Research* 23(6):975–1004.

Rural Aging Roundup [Newsletter published by the National Center on Rural Aging]. 1987. 2(2):1–3.

Rutledge, R., Bell, E., Baker, C. C., and Ricketts, T. C. 1990. *A geographic and statistical analysis of the effects of rural and urban residence on trauma deaths in North Carolina*. Paper presented to the 13th annual meeting of the National Rural Health Association, New Orleans, May 16–19.

Rutter, M. 1987. Psychosocial resilience and protective mechanisms. *American Journal of Orthopsychiatry* 57:316–331.

Rutter, M., Maughan, B., Mortimore, P., and Ouston, T. 1979. *Fifteen thousand hours: Secondary schools and their effects on children.* Cambridge, Massachussets: Harvard University Press.

Sanders, A. B. 1989. Emergency medicine. *Journal of the American Medical Association* 261(19):2841–2843.

Sandrick, K. 1988. U.S. M.D. glut limits demand for FMG physicians. *Hospitals* 62(3):67–69.

Scheer, J., and Groce, N. 1988. Impairment as a human constant: Cross-cultural and historical perspectives on variation. *Journal of Social Issues* 44:23–37.

Schlosberg, J. 1989. The MSA mess. *American Demographics* 10(1):53–58.

Schmelzer, J. R. 1990. *Inter-county variations in Medicare Part B per capita expenditures: Effects of structural, institutional, and socio-economic factors.* Report prepared by the Wisconsin Rural Health Research Center for the Office of Rural Health Policy, HRSA, PHS, DHHS. Marshfield, Wisconsin: Wisconsin Rural Health Research Center.

Schneller, E. S. 1976. The design and evolution of the physician's assistant. *Sociology of Work and Occupations* 3(4):455–478.

Schwartz, W. B., Newhouse, J. P., Bennett, B. W., and Williams, A. P. 1980. The changing geographic distribution of board-certified physicians. *New England Journal of Medicine* 303(18):1032–1038.

Schwartz, W. B., Williams, A. P., Newhouse, J. P., and Witsberger, C. 1988a. Are we training too many medical subspecialists? *Journal of the American Medical Association* 259:233–239.

Schwartz, W. B., Sloan, F. A., and Mendelson, D. N. 1988b. Why there will be little or no physician surplus between now and the year 2000. *New England Journal of Medicine* 318(14):892–897.

Scotch, R. K. 1988. Disability as the basis for a social movement: Advocacy and the politics of definition. *Journal of Social Issues* 44:159–172.

Serow, W. J. 1988. Why the elderly move: Cross-national comparisons. *Research on Aging* 9:582–597.

Shannon, G. W., and Dever, G. E. A. 1974. *Health care delivery: Spatial perspectives.* New York: McGraw-Hill.

Shannon, G. W., Bashshur, R. L., and Metzner, C. A. 1969. The concept of distance as a factor in accessibility and utilization of health care. *Medical Care Review* 26(2):143–161.

Sheps, C. G., and Bachar, M. 1981. Rural areas and personal health services: Current strategies. *American Journal of Public Health.* 71(suppl.): 71–82.

Sheps, C. G., Wagner, E. H., Schonfeld, W. H., DeFriese, G. H., Bachar, M., Brooks, E. F., Gillings, D. B., Guild, P. A, Konrad, T. R., McLaughlin, C. P., Ricketts, T. C., Seipp, C., and Stein, J. S. 1983. An evaluation of subsidized rural primary care programs: I. A typology of practice organizations. *American Journal of Public Health.* 73(1):38–49.

Simmons, H. G. 1982. *From asylum to welfare.* Toronto: National Institute on Mental Retardation.

Simpson, R. J. 1984. *Migrant patterns of the senior population in Southern Ontario.* Toronto: Hemson Consulting.

Sinclair, B., and Manderscheid, L. V. 1974. *A comparative evaluation of indexes of rurality—Their policy implications and distributional impacts.* Research and Development Grant No. 21-26-73-52. Report prepared for the Manpower Administration, U.S. Department of Labor. East Lansing, Michigan: Department of Agricultural Economics, Michigan State University.

Smit, B., and Joseph, A. E. 1984. Identifying service priorities of rural consumers. In *Rural public services: International comparisons*, ed. R. E. Lonsdale and G. Enyedi, pp. 39–49. Boulder, Colorado: Westview.

Smith, B. J., and Parvin, D. W., Jr. 1973. Defining and measuring rurality. *Southern Journal of Agricultural Economics* 5(1):109–113.

Smith, B. W. H., Landick, R., and Dodge, R. 1982. A curricular model for a rural family practice clerkship. *Public Health Reports* 97:373–379.

Smith, C. J. 1988. *Public problems: The management of urban distress.* New York: Guilford Press.

Smith, J. P., Balazs, I. B., Hill, A. S., and Frey, C. F. 1985. Prehospital stabilization of critically injured patients: A failed concept. *Journal of Trauma* 25(1):65–70.

Smith, N. 1987. The incidence of severe trauma in small rural hospitals. *Journal of Family Practice* 25:595–600.

Soldo, B. J., and Agree, E. M. 1988. *America's elderly. Population Bulletin* 43(3).

Sorkin, A. 1986. *Health care and the changing economic environment.* Lexington, Massachussetts: D. C. Heath.

Spaulding, W. B., and Spitzer, W. O. 1972. Implications of medical manpower trends in Ontario 1961–1971. *Ontario Medical Review* September:527–533.

Spears, S. F. 1986. Life threatening emergencies: Patterns of demand and response of a regional emergency medical services system. *American Journal of Preventive Medicine* 2(3):163–168.

Special Committee on Aging, U.S. Senate. 1988. *Staff report: The rural health care challenge.* Serial No. 100-N. Washington, D.C.: U.S. Government Printing Office.

Stambler, H. 1989. Director, Office of Data and Management, Bureau of Health Professions, Health Resources and Services Administration, Public Health Service, U.S. Department of Health and Human Services, Rockville, Maryland. Personal communication, March.

Starr, P. 1981. The politics of therapeutic nihilism. In *The sociology of health and illness: Critical perspectives,* ed. P. Conrad, and R. Kern. New York: St. Martin's Press.

Statistics Canada. 1984. *The elderly in Canada.* Ottawa: Statistics Canada.

———. 1986. *Census of Canada, Census subdivisions and divisions, Ontario, Parts I and II.* Ottawa: Government Printer.

———. 1987. *Canada year book 1988.* Ottawa: Supply and Services Canada.

———. 1988. *The Health and Activity Limitation Survey. Selected data for Canada, provinces, and territories.* Ottawa: Statistics Canada.

———. 1989. *Canada year book 1990.* Ottawa: Supply and Services Canada.

Steinberg, L., Catalano, R., and Dooley, D. 1981. Economic antecedents of child abuse and neglect. *Child Development* 52:975–983.

Stokes, G. 1985. Epidemiological studies of the psychological response to economic instability in England: A summary. In *Health policy implications of unemployment,* ed. G. Wescott, D. P. G. Svensson, and H. F. K. Zollner, pp. 133–142. Copenhagen: World Health Organization.

Stolberg, A. L., Camplair, C., Couvier, K., and Wells, M. J. 1987. Individual, familial, and environmental determinants of children's post-divorce adjustment and maladjustment. *Journal of Divorce* 11:51–70.

Stone, L. E., and Fletcher, S. 1986. *The seniors boom*. Ottawa: Statistics Canada.

Stroman, D. F. 1982. *The awakening minorities. The physically handicapped.* Lanham, Maryland: University Press of America.

Struyk, R., and Soldo, B. 1980. *Improving the elderly's housing. A key to preserving the nation's housing stock and neighborhoods*. New York: Harper & Row.

Studnicki, J., Saywell, R. M., and Wiechetek, W. 1976. Foreign medical graduates and Maryland Medicaid. *New England Journal of Medicine* 294:1153–1157.

Swearingen, C. M., and Perrin, J. M. 1977. Foreign medical graduates in rural primary care: The case of western New York state. *Medical Care* 15(4):331–337.

Taylor, M. G. 1987a. *Health insurance and Canadian public policy: The seven decisions that created the Canadian health insurance system and their outcomes* (Second edition). Montreal: McGill-Queen's University Press.

———. 1987b. The Canadian health-care system: After Medicare. In *Health and Canadian society* (Second edition), ed. D. Coburn, C. D'Arcy, G. M. Torrance, and P. New, pp. 73–101. Toronto: Fitzhenry and Whiteside.

Taylor, M., Dickman, W., and Kane, R. 1973. Medical students' attitudes toward rural practice. *Journal of Medical Education* 48:885–895.

Test, M. A. 1981. Effective community treatment of the chronically mentally ill: What is necessary? *Journal of Social Issues* 37:71–86.

Thomas, G. S. 1989. Micropolitan America. *American Demographics* 11(5): 20–24.

Thrall, G. I., and Tsitanidis, J. G. 1983. A model of the change, attributable to government health insurance plans, in location patterns of physicians—With supporting evidence from Ontario, Canada. *Environment and Planning C: Government and Policy* 1:45–55.

Tiedemann, M. L. 1987. *Educational and curricular factors affecting physician practice location*. Unpublished Ph.D. dissertation, University of Arizona, Tucson.

Tienda, M. 1981. The Mexican-American population. In *Nonmetropolitan America in transition*, ed. A. H. Hawley and S. M. Mazie, pp. 502–550. Chapel Hill, North Carolina: University of North Carolina Press.

Tilson, H., and Jellinek, P. 1981. Primary health care and the local health department: The North Carolina experience. *American Journal of Public Health* 71(suppl.):35–45.

Timpson, J. 1983. An indigenous mental health program in remote Northwestern Ontario: Development and training. *Canada's Mental Health* 31(3): 2, 10.

Todd, A. D. 1984. Women and the disabled in contemporary society. *Social Policy* 14:44–46.

Torrance, G. M. 1987. Socio-historical overview. In *Health and Canadian society* (Second edition), ed. D. Coburn, C. D'Arcy, G. M. Torrance, and P. New, pp. 6–32. Toronto: Fitzhenry and Whiteside.

Trickett, E. J. 1984. Toward a distinctive community psychology: An ecological metaphor for the conduct of community research and the nature of training. *American Journal of Community Psychology* 12:261–279.

Unger, D. G., and Wandersman, A. 1985. The importance of neighbors: The social, cognitive, and affective components of neighboring. *American Journal of Community Psychology* 13:139–169.

University of Arizona College of Medicine Admissions Committee. 1989. *Annual report to the faculty.* Unpublished. Tucson: University of Arizona.

University of North Carolina Health Services Research Center. 1983. *National evaluation of rural primary health care programs: Report to the Robert Wood Johnson Foundation.* Chapel Hill, North Carolina: University of North Carolina Health Services Research Center.

———. 1985. *National evaluation of rural primary health care programs: Supplementary analyses.* Chapel Hill, North Carolina: University of North Carolina Health Services Research Center.

Urdaneta, L. F., Miller, B. K., Ringenberg, B. J., Cram, A. E., and Scott, D. H. 1987. Role of an emergency helicopter transport service in rural trauma. *Archives of Surgery* 122:992–996.

U.S. Congress, House of Representatives. Task Force on the Rural Elderly of the Select Committee on Aging. 1983. *Status of the rural elderly,* Vol. I. Committee Publication No. 98-397. Washington, D.C.: U.S. Government Printing Office.

U.S. Congress, House of Representatives. Committee on Post Office and Civil Service. 1988a. *Designating Morgan and Lawrence Counties in Alabama as a single metropolitan statistical area.* House Report 100-503. Washington, D.C.: U.S. Government Printing Office.

U.S. Congress, House of Representatives. 1988b. Designating Morgan and Lawrence Counties in Alabama as a single metropolitan statistical area. *Congressional Record* 134: March 1 and 2.

U.S. Department of Commerce, Bureau of the Census. 1975. *Historical statistics of the U.S., Colonial times to 1970,* Bicentennial Edition, Part 2. Washington, D.C.: U.S. Government Printing Office.

———. 1980. *Geography for a changing society. Census 80: Continuing Factfinder tradition.* Washington, D.C.: U.S. Government Printing Office.

———. 1981. *Census of Population, 1980,* Vol. 1: *Characteristics of the population: General social and economic characteristics.* Washington, D.C.: U.S. Government Printing Office.

———. 1983a. *Census of population and housing, 1980: Public-use microdata samples, technical documentation.* Washington, D.C.: U.S. Government Printing Office.

———. 1983b. *County and city data book.* Washington, D.C.: U.S. Government Printing Office.

———. 1985. *Census and geography—Concepts and products.* CFF No. 8. Washington, D.C.: U.S. Government Printing Office.

———. 1988. *Statistical abstract of the United States 1988,* 108th Edition. Washington, D.C.: U.S. Government Printing Office.

———. 1991. *Census of population, 1990: Preliminary counts.* Washington, D.C.: U.S. Government Printing Office.

U.S. Department of Commerce, Bureau of the Census, and U.S. Department of Agriculture, Economic Research Service. 1988. *Rural and rural farm population 1987.* Current Population Reports: Farm Population, Series P-27, No. 61. Washington, D.C.: U.S. Government Printing Office.

U.S. Department of Commerce, Office of Federal Statistical Policy and Standards, Federal Committee on Standard Metropolitan Statistical

Areas. 1979. *The metropolitan statistical area classification: 1980 official standards and related documents.* Reprints from *Statistical Reporter.* Washington, D.C.: U.S. Government Printing Office.

———. 1980. *The metropolitan statistical area classification: 1980 official standards and related documents.* Reprints from *Statistical Reporter.* Washington, D.C.: U.S. Government Printing Office.

U.S. Department of Health and Human Services. 1980. *Report of the Graduate Medical Education National Advisory Committee (GMENAC) to the Secretary,* Vols. I–VII. Washington, D.C.: U.S. Government Printing Office.

———. 1985a. *Report of the Secretary's Task Force on Black and Minority Health: Mexican Americans, 1971–1981.* Washington, D.C.: U.S. Government Printing Office.

———. 1985b. *Report of the Secretary's Task Force on Black and Minority Health: Executive summary.* Washington, D.C.: U.S. Government Printing Office.

———. 1986. *A review of health professions' requirements studies.* NTIS Document No. HRP-0906789. Springfield, Virginia: National Technical Information Service.

———. 1989. *Report to Congress: Studies of urban-rural and related geographical adjustments in the Medicare Prospective Payment system.* Washington, D.C.: U.S. Department of Health and Human Services.

U.S. Department of Health and Human Services, Bureau of Health Professions. 1983. *The impact of foreign-trained doctors on the supply of physicians.* DHHS No. HRS-P-OD-83-2. Washington, D.C.: U.S. Government Printing Office.

———. 1984. *Evaluation of the effects of National Health Service Corps physician placements upon medical care delivery in rural areas: Non-technical summary.* ODAM Report No. 7-84. Hyattsville, Maryland: Bureau of Health Professions.

———. 1986a. *Young physicians in rural areas: The impact of service in the National Health Service Corps,* Vol. 1: *County characteristics.* ODAM Report No. 3-86. Hyattsville, Maryland: Bureau of Health Professions.

———. 1986b. *Young physicians in rural areas: The impact of service in the National Health Service Corps,* Vol. 2: *Survey of factors influencing the location decision and practice patterns.* ODAM Report No. 4-86. Hyattsville, Maryland: Bureau of Health Professions.

U.S. Department of Health and Human Services, Public Health Service, Health Resources and Services Administration, Bureau of Health Care Delivery and Assistance. 1986. *Primary care activities in frontier areas—Regional Program Guidance Memorandum 86-10.* Unpublished memorandum.

U.S. Department of Health and Human Services, Public Health Service, National Institutes of Health. 1987. *Atlas of U.S. cancer mortality among whites: 1950–1980.* DHHS Publication No. (NIH) 87-2900. Bethesda, Maryland: National Institutes of Health.

U.S. Department of Health and Human Services, Public Health Service, Health Resources and Services Administration, Bureau of Health Professions, Office of Data Analysis. 1988. *The Area Resource File (ARF) System: Information for Health Resources Planning and Research.* ODAM Report No. 6-88. Springfield, Virginia: National Technical Information Service.

U.S. Executive Office of the President, Office of Management and Budget. 1983–1988. Bulletins revising definitions and designations of MSAs, Nos. 83-20, 84-16, 84-24, 85-18, 86-14, and 88-14 (June 27, 1983; June 29, 1984; October 23, 1984; June 27, 1985; June 13, 1986; November 19, 1986; and June 23, 1988). Washington, D.C.: U.S. Government Printing Office.

U.S. General Accounting Office. 1989. *Medicare Catastrophic Act. Options for changing financing and benefits.* Report to the Chairman, Committee on Ways and Means, House of Representatives. Washington, D.C.: U.S. Government Printing Office.

———. 1991. *Trauma care: Lifesaving system threatened by unreimbursed costs and other factors.* HRD-91-57. Washington, D.C.: U.S. Government Printing Office.

U.S. Health Care Financing Administration. 1985. *Out-of-pocket health expenses for Medicaid recipients and other low-income persons, 1980. National Medical Care Utilization and Expenditure Survey.* Series B, Descriptive Report No. 4. Baltimore, Maryland: Health Care Financing Administration.

U.S. National Center for Health Statistics. 1984. National Health Interview Survey. In *Health, United States, 1983.* DHHS (PHS) 84-1232. Washington, D.C.: U.S. Government Printing Office.

———. 1986a. *Current estimates from the National Health Interview Survey, 1985.* Series 10.160. Washington, D.C.: U.S. Government Printing Office.

———. 1986b. *Current estimates from the National Health Interview Survey, 1984.* Series 10.156. Washington, D.C.: U.S. Government Printing Office.

———. 1989. Advance report of final mortality statistics, 1987. *Monthly Vital Statistics Report* 38(5).

Verby, J. 1988. The Minnesota rural physician associate program. *Journal of Medical Education* 63:427–437.

Wachs, M. 1979. *Transportation for the elderly. Changing lifestyles, changing needs.* Berkeley and Los Angeles: University of California Press.

Wallace, R., Macdonald, J. R., and Rose, A. 1984. *Factors affecting the quality of life of community-based elderly,* Part I: *Literature review.* Research Paper No. 151. Toronto: Centre for Urban and Community Studies, University of Toronto.

Waller, J. A. 1974. The smaller hospital in the health care system. A rural EMS categorization system. *Hospitals* 48(19)111–112, 114, 116.

Waller, J. A., Garner, R., and Lawrence, R. 1966. Utilization of ambulance services in a rural community. *American Journal of Public Health* 56(3): 513–520.

Watkins, H. E., and Bradbard, M. R. 1982. Child maltreatment: An overview with suggestions for intervention and research. *Family Relations* 21:323–333.

Wayne, R. 1989. Rural trauma management. *American Journal of Surgery* 157:463–467.

Wears, R. L. 1989. Predicting the demand for "emergency" medical services. *Annals of Emergency Medicine* 18(6):705–706.

Weaver, C. L. 1986. Social security disability policy in the 1980s and beyond. In *Disability and the labor market. Economic problems, policies, and programs,* ed. M. Berkowitz and M. A. Hill, pp. 29–63. Ithaca, New York: Cornell University Press.

Weiss, J. E., Greenlick, M. R., and Jones, J. F. 1971. Determinants of medical care utilization: The impact of spatial factors. *Inquiry* 8(1):50–57.

West, M., Mennin, S. P., Kaufman, A., and Galey, W. 1982. Medical students' attitudes toward basic sciences: Influence of a primary care curriculum. *Medical Education* 16(4):188–191.

Wilkens, R., and Adams, O. B. 1987. Health expectancy in Canada, late 1970s. In *Health and Canadian society* (Second edition), ed. D. Coburn, C. D'Arcy, G. M. Torrance, and P. New, pp. 36–56. Toronto: Fitzhenry and Whiteside.

Williams, R. 1973. *The country and the city.* Oxford: Oxford University Press.

Williams, R., and Chen, P. 1982. Identifying the sources of the recent decline in perinatal mortality rate in California. *New England Journal of Medicine* 306:207–214.

Williams, A. P., Schwartz, W. B., Newhouse, J. P., and Bennett, B. W. 1983. How many miles to the doctor? *New England Journal of Medicine* 309: 958–963.

Wilson, S. R. 1979. *An analytical study of physicians' career decisions regarding geographic location. Digest of the final report.* American Institutes for Research, DHEW Contract No. HRA231-77-088. Hyattsville, Maryland: Health Resources Administration, Department of Health, Education and Welfare.

Wimberly, R. C. 1986. Agricultural and rural transition. In *New dimensions in rural policy: Building upon our heritage*, Subcommittee on Agriculture and Transportation, Congress of the United States, pp. 39–45. Washington, D.C.: U.S. Government Printing Office.

Windley, P. G., and Scheidt, R. J. 1988. Rural small towns: An environmental context for aging. *Journal of Rural Studies* 4:151–158.

Wiseman, R. F. 1980. Why older people move. *Research on Aging* 2:141–154.

Wiseman, R. F., and Roseman, C. R. 1979. A typology of elderly migration based on the decision-making process. *Economic Geography* 55:324–337.

Wolfe, D. A. 1987. *Child abuse.* Newbury Park, California: Sage.

Wolfe, J. 1984. The provision of essential services in rural Ontario, Canada. In *Rural public services: International comparisons*, ed. R. E. Lonsdale and G. Enyedi, pp. 85–103. Boulder, Colorado: Westview.

Wunderman, L. E., and Steiber, S. R. 1983. Physicians who move and why. *Journal of Medical Education* 58:389–394.

Yett, D. C., Der, W., Ernst, R. L., and Hay, J. W. 1983. Physician pricing and health insurance reimbursement. *Health Care Financing Review* 5(2):69–80.

Yett, D. C., and Sloan, F. A. 1974. Migration patterns of recent medical school graduates. *Inquiry* 11:125–142.

Young, T. K. 1987. The health of Indians in northwestern Ontario. In *Health and Canadian society* (Second edition), ed. D. Coburn, C. D'Arcy, G. M. Torrance, and P. New, pp. 109–126. Toronto: Fitzhenry and Whiteside.

Zapf, M. 1985. *Rural social work and its applications to the Canadian north as a practice setting.* Toronto: University of Toronto Press.

Index